T0200168

Community Child
and Adolescent Psychiatry
A Manual of Clinical Practice and Consultation

Community Child
and Adolescent Psychiatry
A Manual of Clinical Practice and Consultation

Edited by

Theodore A. Petti, M.D., M.P.H.

Carlos Salguero, M.D., M.P.H.

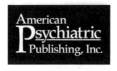

Washington, DC
London, England

Note: The authors have worked to ensure that all information in this book is accurate at the time of publication and consistent with general psychiatric and medical standards, and that information concerning drug dosages, schedules, and routes of administration is accurate at the time of publication and consistent with standards set by the U.S. Food and Drug Administration and the general medical community. As medical research and practice continue to advance, however, therapeutic standards may change. Moreover, specific situations may require a specific therapeutic response not included in this book. For these reasons and because human and mechanical errors sometimes occur, we recommend that readers follow the advice of physicians directly involved in their care or the care of a member of their family.

Books published by American Psychiatric Publishing, Inc. (APPI), represent the views and opinions of the individual authors and do not necessarily represent the policies and opinions of APPI or the American Psychiatric Association.

Copyright © 2006 American Psychiatric Publishing, Inc.
ALL RIGHTS RESERVED
Manufactured in the United States of America on acid-free paper
09 08 07 06 05   5 4 3 2 1
First Edition
Typeset in Bailey Sans ITC and Baskerville Book
American Psychiatric Publishing, Inc.
1000 Wilson Boulevard
Arlington, VA 22209-3901
www.appi.org

Library of Congress Cataloging-in-Publication Data
Community child and adolescent psychiatry : a manual of clinical practice and consultation / [edited] by Theodore A. Petti, Carlos Salguero.—1st ed.
    p. ; cm.
Includes bibliographical references and index.
ISBN 1-58562-180-3 (pbk. : alk. paper)
    1. Child psychiatry. 2. Child mental health services. 3. Community psychiatry. 4. Community mental health services. 5. Adolescent psychiatry.
    [DNLM: 1. Community Mental Health Services—Adolescent.
2. Community Mental Health Services—Child. 3. Community Psychiatry—Adolescent. 4. Community Psychiatry—Child.] I. Petti, Theodore A. II. Salguero, Carlos, 1939–
RJ499.C5965 2005
618.92'89–dc22

                                                                  2005002350

British Library Cataloguing in Publication Data
A CIP record is available from the British Library.

This book is dedicated to the contributors
who stayed with us through the long, tedious process
and to fellow professionals who have and will dedicate
their careers, time, and efforts
in working in the public community sector.
To you we express our gratitude.

And to the American Academy
of Child and Adolescent Psychiatry,
most specifically the Campaign for Children,
to which the proceeds generated from this book will be donated.

To my wife, Mary Newman Petti,
and to the trainees and colleagues who have taught me so much.
T.A.P.

To my wife Susan and my children
and to the children at the Hill Health Center and the Village.
C.S.

CONTENTS

Part I
Principles of Community Practice

Part II

The Core Mental Health Professionals

Part III

Interdisciplinary Functioning in the Community Setting

Part IV

Outcomes and Future
Directions

CONTRIBUTORS

Kathleen E. Albus, Ph.D.
Psychologist, Center for Promotion of Child Development Through Primary Care, Baltimore, Maryland

Valerie Arnold, M.D.
Assistant Professor, Department of Child Psychiatry, University of Tennessee Health Science Center, Memphis, Tennessee

Tanya N. Bryant, B.S.
Program Management Specialist, Center for School Mental Health Assistance, University of Maryland School of Medicine, Baltimore, Maryland

Lance D. Clawson, M.D., F.A.A.C.A.P.
Private Practice, Child and Adolescent Psychiatry, Cabin John, Maryland

Peter R. Cohen, M.D.
Medical Director, Maryland Alcohol and Drug Abuse Administration, Catonsville, Maryland

Stuart Copans, M.D.
Adjunct Associate Professor, Department of Psychiatry, Dartmouth Medical School, Lebanon, New Hampshire; Associate, Departments of Psychiatry and Family Medicine, University of Massachusetts Medical School, Worcester, Massachusetts

Brenda L. Costello-Wells, R.N., M.S.N., C.S.
Advance Practice Nurse, Child and Adolescent Psychiatry, Behavior Corp, Carmel, Indiana

John M. Diamond, M.D.
Professor and Section Head Division of Child and Adolescent Psychiatry, Brody School of Medicine at East Carolina University, Greenville, North Carolina

Judith Dogin, M.D.
Clinical Associate Professor of Psychiatry, Department of Psychiatry, University of Pennsylvania, Philadelphia, Pennsylvania

Theodore Fallon, M.D., M.P.H.
Private Practice, Chester Springs, Pennsylvania

Milton T. Fujita, M.D., M.H.A.
Medical Director, Community Treatment, Inc., Arnold, Missouri; Assistant Clinical Professor, Department of Psychiatry, St. Louis University School of Medicine, St. Louis, Missouri; Assistant Clinical Professor, Psychiatry, Missouri Institute of Psychiatry, University of Missouri-Columbia School of Medicine, Columbia, Missouri

Claire Griffin-Francell, C.N.S./P.M.H., M.S.N.
President, Southeast Nurse Consultants, Atlanta, Georgia

Jerry D. Heston, M.D.
Child and Adolescent Psychiatry Associates, Cordova, Tennessee; Formerly Professor, Department of Psychiatry, University of Tennessee Health Science Center, Memphis, Tennessee

John R. Holmberg, Psy.D.
Senior Instructor, Prevention Research Center for Family and Child Health, University of Colorado, Denver, Colorado

Charles Huffine, M.D.
Clinical Assistant Professor of Psychology and Psychiatry, University of Washington; Medical Director for Child and Adolescent Services, King County Mental Health, Chemical Abuse and Dependency Services Division; Consultant to Youth Advocates, Seattle, Washington

Charles Keith, M.D.
Associate Professor of Psychiatry (retired), Division of Child and Adolescent Psychiatry, Department of Psychiatry, Duke University Medical Center, Durham, North Carolina

Laurel J. Kiser, Ph.D., M.B.A.
Associate Professor, Department of Psychiatry, University of Maryland, Baltimore, Maryland

Richard J. Lawlor, Ph.D., J.D.
Associate Professor of Psychiatry and Chief, Forensic Psychiatry Services, Indiana University School of Medicine, Indianapolis, Indiana

Alice Long, M.A.
Director, Therapeutic Preschool Consultant, Operation Breakthrough Head Start, Division of Child and Adolescent Psychiatry, Department of Psychiatry, Duke University Medical Center, Durham, North Carolina

Laura A. Nabors, Ph.D.
Assistant Professor, Department of Psychology, University of Cincinnati, Cincinnati, Ohio

Peter Nierman, M.D.
Assistant Professor, Child and Adolescent Psychiatry, Institute for Juvenile Research, University of Illinois–Chicago, Department of Psychiatry; Network Manager for Metro C & A Network, Chicago, Illinois

Nancy D. Opie, R.N., D.N.S., F.A.A.N.
Professor Emeritus, Department of Environments for Health, Indiana University School of Nursing, Indianapolis, Indiana

Marilyn Paavola, L.C.S.W.
Child and Adolescent Psychiatry Associates, Cordova, Tennessee; Formerly Instructor, Department of Psychiatry, University of Tennessee Health Science Center, Memphis, Tennessee

Dean X. Parmelee, M.D.
Associate Dean for Academic Affairs, Professor of Psychiatry and Pediatrics, Wright State University School of Medicine, Dayton, Ohio

Theodore A. Petti, M.D., M.P.H.
Professor of Psychiatry and Director, Division of Child and Adolescent Psychiatry, Robert Wood Johnson Medical School–University of Medicine and Dentistry of New Jersey, Piscataway, New Jersey

Frances S. Porter, A.C.S.W., L.C.S.W.
Former Director, Casey Family Services, Hartford Division, Hartford, Connecticut

John Ronnau, Ph.D., A.C.S.W.
Vice President for Administration and Partnership Affairs, The University of Texas Brownsville and Texas Southmost College, Brownsville, Texas

Carlos Salguero, M.D., M.P.H., F.A.P.A.
Medical Director Village for Families and Children, Hartford, Connecticut; Associate Clinical Professor of Pediatrics and Psychiatry, Yale Child Study Center, New Haven, Connecticut

Donna S. Vitulano, M.S.W.
Research Associate, Child Study Center, Yale School of Medicine, New Haven, Connecticut; Social Work Site Coordinator, Bridgeport Health Department, Bridgeport, Connecticut

Lawrence A. Vitulano, Ph.D.
Associate Clinical Professor, Child Study Center, Yale School of Medicine, New Haven, Connecticut

Mark D. Weist, Ph.D.
Professor, Department of Psychiatry, University of Maryland School of Medicine, Baltimore, Maryland

INTRODUCTION

These are exciting times for those in child psychiatry and related fields. During the Decade of the Brain, advances were made in the care and treatment of mentally ill children and teenagers. In response to the reported excesses of institutional care, pediatric mental health professionals are placing greater focus on community-based services. This manual is a guide for child psychiatrists, child psychologists, clinical nurses, social workers, and other mental health practitioners working in community settings. It is the practice component of a manual developed by the Committee on Community Psychiatry and Consultation to Agencies of the American Academy of Child and Adolescent Psychiatry. Day-to-day concerns of professionals working on behalf of children and adolescents in community settings predominantly served by or in conjunction with the public sector are the focus. Confronted daily with a plethora of conflicts, crises, and dilemmas, such professionals—consultants, staff members, and administrators in community agencies—struggle with issues that are compounded by the nature of the public sector: limited funds, the poverty and adversarial social environments in which many of the families served live, and the nature of bureaucracies within which public agencies are embedded.

These professionals have a tremendous impact on individual children, on families, and on the greater community. They have access to and are able to utilize resources that are not available to those in private practice. Professionals entering the public-sector arena often have little guidance and lack a comparative standard to facilitate their work. It is our hope that readers who turn to this manual for answers will find approaches or insights that will make their work easier or will help them be more productive. The manual provides a road map to a higher level of practice in community settings. For trainees in child and adolescent psychiatry, it furnishes an overview of expected levels of practice and a concrete approach to the ambiguous situations that are characteristic of community and consultation issues. For professionals from the traditional mental health disciplines, it is a guide to what to expect from colleagues in other disciplines. For administrators, it can serve as a guide to deploying relatively scarce resources. Readers will find explicit descriptions of the direct and indirect tasks, strategies, and maneuvers that child- and family-focused community mental health professionals can choose to consider. By employing these methods, readers should be able to function more effectively in community systems and agencies.

Questions the mental health professional must consider before assuming a staff or administrative position in a community agency are addressed from numerous perspectives. We hope readers will learn to work more effectively and to position themselves to experience the joys, opportunities, and sense of satisfaction that community practice can provide, while avoiding the pitfalls inherent in working for public-sector agencies. Legal and ethical issues pertaining to particular agencies are also presented. A multidisciplinary environment has become increasingly important in contemporary community psychiatry. The manual assists readers in considering reasonable roles for various disciplines and team members. For professionals entering into community work, either as consultants or in the delivery of direct services, the manual provides an overview of general principles for working in the public sector and tools to assess the sector in which professionals plan to work; the general issues that representative agencies are likely to present; and the overall mission of particular types of agencies. Potential opportunities for readers to make significant contributions to the health and welfare of the families under their care, their agencies, and their communities are highlighted.

Introductory chapters address the particular nature of working in or consulting to community agencies from the perspectives of major mental health disciplines employed in community settings. Basic principles of community practice are emphasized, and the dynamics and characteristics of issues commonly faced by public-sector professionals are discussed. Differences between rural and urban practice are addressed. In later chapters, these principles are discussed as they apply to particular types of agencies. Efforts are made to consider contemporary concern about the impact of a managed care or a cost-cutting environment on service delivery. Keeping current in a rapidly changing world, handling reimbursement, differentiating between consultation and direct service, and finding one's place in a system of care are addressed. Each chapter addressing a type of community agency begins with a description of the setting or activity and then elaborates on the salient features that would allow a professional or trainee to enter and work in that system with more confidence than he or she would have after reading a textbook or attending a lecture. Practicalities of clinical practice or consultation in community settings in the current service environment are depicted. The manual presents consultation to those same agencies from different perspectives. Steps or phases of the consultation are described, and special consideration is given to different types of demands. Professionals wishing to begin a consultative practice or to improve their current consultative activities will find many practical facts and insights to guide them in those endeavors.

Guidance is provided for situations when child mental health clinicians or administrators find that their roles as consultant, staff member, or administrator are blurred. The manual provides descriptions of how to blend these tasks and lays out explicit, basic rules. Where consultation from child mental health professionals may be of value is illustrated. We hope this manual will serve as a ready reference for difficult or unanticipated situations. This is a practice manual, not a textbook, and hence references and a literature review are included only as absolutely needed. The emphasis is on the practical necessities of child psychiatrists and other professionals working with mentally ill youngsters and their families in the practice of community psychiatry and public mental health care. The manual is also intended to aid professionals engaged in the private sector who wish to understand the functioning and dynamics of the public sector and who are seeking opportunities to participate in the evolution of community mental health practice.

Each chapter presents the perspectives of seasoned clinicians and administrators who have a wide and practical grasp of their area of expertise. Overlap in critical areas occurs between chapters and provides readers with alternative views of similar issues. A full reading of each chapter will provide the panorama needed to understand the complexity and richness afforded by the public mental health sector and the opportunities to do good work. Gems of information in one chapter will round out the discussion addressed differently in other chapters. Special attention is not devoted to the area of systems of care because the topic is comprehensively addressed in a related publication (Pumariega and Winters 2003).

Functional and effective arrays of community services are evolving in the public sector to address the needs of disturbed youngsters with severe and persistent mental illness (i.e., chronically ill youths) and are of particular importance for mentally ill youngsters and their families. Training of mental health professionals has been uneven in this area. Inadequate understanding of the structure and process of community systems and agencies is common. Managed care and its antecedents have dramatically altered the service-system landscape, especially in the private sector but increasingly in the community arena. Blending of funds, decategorization, wraparound services, outcome measurement, continuum of care, and cultural sensitivity are all newly minted icons of basic principles that have long been known and at one time or another actively espoused.

With the practical applications of this manual in mind, it is useful to consider community mental health from a historical perspective. As noted by Levine and Levine (1992), from the late nineteenth century to the early part of the twentieth century, a preventive orientation in community mental health was prevalent. Early child guidance clinics worked with public schools, but by the 1960s child guidance clinics had minimal contact with the schools regarding children they were assessing or treating. Most core mental health professionals working in the public sector were found in child guidance and related clinics. In 1963, President John F. Kennedy signed the Community Mental Health Centers (CMHCs) Act (P.L. 88-164) into law. In 1970, Congress modified it to include children among the groups that the centers are required to serve. Some child guidance clinics became incorporated into CMHCs to provide that component.

The thrust toward consultation increased involvement by schools. However, restrictions on confidentiality limited two-way communication. The preventive orientation model was supplanted by treatment of individual children from an intrapsychic or personal weakness mode, which moved away from the mode in which the environment was seen as being in need of change. Society is moving again toward involving community agencies in helping youngsters with significant psychiatric disorders. *Helping Children: A Social History* (Levine and Levine 1992) is essential reading for understanding some of these changes and the context in which they occurred.

Jane Knitzer's 1982 book *Unclaimed Children* highlighted a governmental lack of commitment to provide services, lack of advocacy for children, and lack of policy direction. In response, in 1984 the National Institute of Mental Health created the Child and Adolescent Service System Program (CASSP). The mission of CASSP was to assist states and communities in developing systems of care for children and youths with serious emotional problems and for the families of these children.

The principles of CASSP brought a new conceptual framework in which a child was seen in the context of a coordinated system of care. This framework has led to expanded children's mental health services that have widely benefited the public sector; the private sector seems to be applying similar principles through managed care and related organizations. These principles, described in several chapters of the manual, essentially involve development and implementation of child-centered services—focused on the family within a community base—that are expected to meet the individual child's needs by recognizing and addressing cultural and related issues.

To address the difficulty of serving children and adolescents with serious emotional disturbance (SED), multiple approaches and systems have been either suggested or implemented since CASSP's inception. Fragmentation of services resulting from categorization of funds to particular agencies serving the same youngsters was recognized as a major barrier. The Robert Wood Johnson Foundation initiated a program to serve youngsters with SED in a family-centered, cost-effective manner (i.e., a family-focused, community-based, capitated managed care system of services for children with SED and their families). Projects were to be consumer oriented and accountable for outcomes and were to maximally use all funding sources. Blending of resources from child-serving agencies was the goal, so that funding would be decategorized to eliminate artificial barriers for funding allocated for specific categories of need. This approach, which has been described under numerous labels (such as wraparound services and multisystemic therapy), adheres to the principles and values of CASSP (Burns et al. 2000). Advances evolving from these initiatives and the ways that community mental health will be practiced in the new millennium will reflect the influence of this program. Parallel advances have occurred in school-based health centers, many with a mental health component. Yet significant proportions of the most vulnerable populations in poor, violent, drug-ridden inner cities and in poverty-ridden rural areas have difficulty gaining access to needed services. Likewise, the 2000 annual report of the federally funded Coalition for Juvenile Justice reported that a substantial majority of incarcerated children and adolescents and those in juvenile detention centers have unmet mental health needs (http://www.juvjustice.org).

This manual provides readers with insight into the public system of care and the requisite tools to manage the rapidly changing clinical, political, and administrative landscape. Several books describe aspects of the community system (Fritz et al. 1993; Ghuman and Sarles 1998; Pumariega and Winters 2003) across the spectrum. Our manual links those efforts from the perspective of academic centers to provide a concise reference encompassing a wider swath of community mental health practice. We hope that readers find the book useful and stimulating.

Theodore A. Petti, M.D., M.P.H.
Carlos Salguero, M.D., M.P.H.

▎ REFERENCES

Burns BJ, Schoenwald SK, Burchard JD, et al: Comprehensive community-based interventions for youth with severe emotional disorders: multisystemic therapy and the wraparound process. J Child Fam Stud 9:283–314, 2000

Community Mental Health Centers Act of 1963, Pub. L. No. 88-164

Fritz GK, Mattison RE, Nurcombe B, et al: Child and Adolescent Mental Health Consultation in Hospitals, Schools, and Courts. Washington, DC, American Psychiatric Press, 1993

Ghuman HS, Sarles RM: Handbook of Child and Adolescent Outpatient, Day Treatment and Community Psychiatry. Philadelphia, PA, Brunner/Mazel, 1998

Knitzer J: Unclaimed Children: The Failure of Public Responsibility to Children and Adolescents in Need of Mental Health Services. Washington, DC, Children's Defense Fund, 1982

Levine ML, Levine A: Helping Children: A Social History. New York, Oxford University Press, 1992

Pumariega AJ, Winters NC (eds): The Handbook of Child and Adolescent Systems of Care: The New Community Psychiatry. San Francisco, CA, Jossey-Bass, 2003

PART

I

Principles of Community Practice

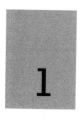

WORKING WITHIN COMMUNITIES

Theodore A. Petti, M.D., M.P.H.

This chapter provides an overview of two critical areas of community child and adolescent mental health work: 1) clinical practice and administration and 2) consultation to community agencies. Communities are social groups of individuals living in some proximity to each other to share services and to provide security and physical safety. Community mental health workers (CMHWs) are professional, paraprofessional, or allied health persons who employ mental health training and experience within a shared system of human services. Most CMHWs wear many hats, with differing roles depending on their administrative and clinical responsibilities or situation and depending on the structure and setting of the community agency or network that determines the role, responsibilities, functions, and limitations of the position. A kaleidoscopic CMHW role is inherent in systems, with blurred roles and functions being typical in human service organizations. Practice or providing consultation is certainly more complex in some communities or agencies than in others.

∎ CLINICAL PRACTICE AND ADMINISTRATION

Characterization of Community Agencies

CMHWs are generally employed by human service agencies (HSAs): health and mental health centers, schools, juvenile courts, and welfare agencies. Mental health professionals working in or consulting for community programs must become aware of essential features of the agency (e.g., the degree of environmental support and whether the structure and culture of the agency fit and sustain its purposes). Major organizational features include the following (Weisbord 1978):

- *Goals:* 1) The degree to which the aims of the agency are clearly stated and understood, and 2) the level of commitment to those aims by members of the agency or network.
- *Structure:* Interdependence between and within agency components, including formal mechanisms (e.g., organizational charts) and informal mechanisms (e.g., gatherings around coffee machines) that facilitate completion of work.
- *Interrelations:* Interpersonal, intergroup, and interactive relationships that determine within-agency conflict management and dissemination of practice advances (e.g., policy development and implementation in a multidisciplinary agency with financial support for different projects of equal priority).
- *Reward for productivity:* Outcomes to determine accountability. The goals and purposes of most HSAs are poorly defined. With scarce financial resources, reward options may be limited to promotion, enhanced job titles, social recognition, and additional responsibilities. Determining workers' perceptions of the reinforcement schedule and how that schedule compares to public description of rewards, sanctions, and risk taking is critical.
- *Leadership style:* How well the other five areas function together, which indicates the extent to which the leadership is able to define, embody, and defend the organization's purposes and effectively manage conflict.
- *Helping mechanisms:* Features that allow organizations to maintain their culture (e.g., newsletters, bulletins, e-mails, work groups) and support other functions.

A helpful mnemonic is G SIR LEADS HELP'M:

G	Goals
SIR	Structure, Interrelations, Reward for productivity
LEADS	Leadership
HELP'M	Helping mechanisms

CMHWs should review these factors before joining and before deciding to remain in or leave a particular community HSA and while assessing a commitment to engage in community activity. The compatibility of one's personal style and approaches with agency culture and functioning is critical in determining the likelihood of workplace success and satisfaction and is important when considering entering into public- or community-sector work.

HSAs generally have the following characteristics (Goodstein 1983):

- They operate as if clients have a single, isolated problem that can be solved by the agency autonomously.
- They are problem oriented rather than person oriented.
- Their clients are responsible for creating links to other services.
- Their clients count on bureaucratic competence to work for them.
- There is a lack of interdependence between agencies.
- Agency survival is not dependent on "success."
- Conflict is managed by smoothing over differences.
- There is an emphasis on autonomous exercise of skill and professional behavior.
- The hurts from confronting an issue are healed through careful preparation and follow-up.
- There is an emphasis on facilitating communication and referral to reduce interagency boundaries (i.e., communication and coordination take precedence over integration and consolidation).

Gaining an understanding of the general characteristics and dynamics of a system in which one is employed as a staff member, administrator, or consultant may allow one to feel involved, needed, productive, and satisfied. Failing to attend to these issues increases the risk of personalizing the adverse occurrences and situations that are common in community settings, thus raising the risk of burnout and ultimate departure from the agency or public-sector arena.

The roles that are filled by mental health professionals within community agencies have required modifications to existing mental health practice models. Most CMHWs typically serve many functions in community agencies and find themselves blending multiple roles within the same organization in adapting to the realities of managed care and school-based services.

Practice in Community Agencies

Roles and Conflicts of CMHWs

For CMHWs, practice in an HSA involves occupying a designated position in the agency's organizational chart; relating to a supervisor, administrator, or governing board; and playing a role within the organizational structure. Practitioners of all clinical disciplines have served as administrators and supervisors as well as staff members within agencies. Professional roles are defined by the degree of authority and responsibility exercised within the organization. Staff members within HSA structures must function with and relate (at various levels depending on the staff member's position) to the board or governing body, administrators, supervisors, and coworkers and must also interact with the external environment. The dichotomy between professional and staff roles of CMHWs has become blurred in some respects and sharpened perceptibly in others. Professionals are much less free to practice as their professional organizations suggest or recommend. Requests for CMHWs to apply critical-pathway guidelines, to follow administrative dictums related to practice, and to ally themselves much closer to their agency than to their professional associations partially account for this clouding of role definitions as economists and planners seek interchangeable units of service at the least cost to society and the organization. Before accepting a staff or administrative position with an HSA, mental health professionals must consider the basic characteristics of HSAs and the factors of general responsibility outlined in the subsections that follow.

Administrative Responsibility

Administrative responsibility has traditionally been awarded or assigned to clinical staff members working their way up the hierarchy to middle and upper management in community mental health centers (CMHCs) and other HSAs. As more funds flowed into those systems and fiscal issues became increasingly important, professional managers eventually began to assume those positions. However, clinicians frequently remain in major agency positions. Those aspiring to administrative positions should develop skills for blending clinical and administrative duties. At the highest agency levels, administrative responsibility involves developing and implementing policy, relating to the governing or advisory board, and interacting with outside agencies. At the clinical care level, accountability includes accepting responsibility and exercising authority to supervise the delivery of the highest appropriate level of care by considering the clinical needs of the child and family commensurate with safety for the community and within the bounds of available funding for services at the particular agency or community system.

Clinical Responsibility

Clinical responsibility involves the range of direct services or supervision of care—that is, accountability in legal and fiscal areas and staff-related education and training. Authority coupled with responsibility allows the community practitioner to be effective. Absence of authority creates a risky situation for the clinician or clinical administrator. The combination of high clinical supervisory responsibility and low authority to make and implement decisions creates a recipe for frustration and ineffective functioning. Care of the individual patient or family tempered by overall community and agency needs and resources is a balance toward which the clinician and clinical supervisor must strive.

Administrative and clinical responsibilities overlap considerably for senior clinicians. For example, when caring for youngsters with disruptive disorders, with compulsive disorders involving stealing or fire setting, or with psychotic behavior, situations can arise that may place the youngster, the family, and society at risk:

> Dr. M, a child and adolescent psychiatrist who is employed as a consultant to a CMHC, is presented with a 7-year-old fire setter who was seen briefly by the intake worker and was evaluated in a 1-hour session by a master's-level clinician. Dr. M is asked to sign off on the evaluation and diagnosis. The managed care organization (MCO) insists that one evaluation session is sufficient for outpatient care.

This case illustrates dilemmas faced by one particular discipline. Psychiatrists must make decisions regarding the exigencies of limited resources, perceived turf issues with other clinicians, and externally placed restrictions on clinical practice versus their own preparatory training and minimum standards of practice designated by professional organizations. This situation forces psychiatrists to choose between risking noncompliance with the professional and ethical standards of their discipline versus purportedly endangering the financial well-being of the agency that pays their salary.

Care for individual children and their families is in danger of being left out of the equation. In the case outlined above, the psychiatrist or psychologist might not make a diagnosis for treatment planning after a single session and would be leery of such a diagnosis made by a less experienced person. Yet the exigencies of managed behavioral health care demand new ways of conceptualizing and conducting one's clinical practice—for example, employing standardized self-report instruments to gather data usually obtained through the clinical interview. Similar problems can occur with Medicaid reimbursement and when CMHCs fail to contract for sufficient psychiatric and other professional time for adequate assessment and treatment. The potential to underutilize CMHWs through questionable superspecialization and restriction of practice is worrisome. Professional staff members are responsible to the agency and its governing body for their actions and for the profit, loss, or liability resulting from their decisions or actions. The constriction of the scope of practice for CMHWs can become problematic for fiscal, moral, and ethical reasons and can have adverse effects on the morale and sense of identity within the HSA and the community.

An operational structure to facilitate adequate documentation for insurance, disability recommendations, and forensic evaluations is crucial to the overall functioning of the agency and to the effective use of clinical services. Responsibility for ensuring the optimal use of resources within an agency or program is often implicit rather than explicit. CMHWs generally want to provide for the child's needs regardless of the payer system or the socioeconomic status of the family. In the current political environment, CMHWs must learn about the community system and understand legislative, judicial, and executive barriers to (or supports for) appropriate care as outlined in Chapter 2, "Public-Sector Dynamics for Child Mental Health." Knowing how and when to access funding and supporting community resources for an individual child or family (e.g., the Medicaid rehabilitation waiver; Title XX funds; Individuals With Disabilities Education Act, P.L. 101-476) is critically important.

Professional CMHWs have multiple sources for keeping abreast of ongoing changes—for example, professional society newsletters, journals, and meetings; the Internet; and government publications. Besides maintaining knowledge of current administrative issues, clinical supervisors must be aware of the evolving nature of the various models for individual, group, and family psychotherapy (including manual-driven innovations); psychotropic medication; and quality improvement efforts. Doing so and ensuring that other professional and nonprofessional staff members maintain and improve their skills become a real challenge to clinical supervisors and agency staff.

Legal Responsibility

Legal responsibility comprises issues more fully detailed in Chapter 3, "Legal Issues." Clinical and administrative leaders must keep abreast of developments and trends and must ensure that the frontline clinical, clerical, and administrative staff are kept current with recent developments. Familiarity with legal language and jargon facilitates program implementation and maintenance. Understanding contracts and government regulations (e.g., the Health Insurance Portability and Accountability Act of 1996) allows ease in planning, monitoring, information sharing, sustaining communication, and maintaining commitment to the program.

Fiscal Responsibility

Fiscal responsibility is important for clinical and administrative professional staff across all agency levels. Clinicians and administrators are responsible for understanding budgets, legislative and regulatory procedures that can affect the ability to obtain funding and to charge for services, and the mechanisms of collections and related functions. Knowing which forms to complete and how to complete them correctly is of premium value. With expanding regulations and multiple payer sources, incorrect billing or charges can potentially lead to civil and criminal penalties. Seminars, symposia, and workshops abound and are regularly available to assist in developing or maintaining competence in this area.

Education and Training

Education and training of frontline clinical and clerical staff are critical responsibilities. Rapid changes in rules and regulations; research advances in clinical care; and changes in funding, safety codes, accreditation standards, fiscal imperatives, personnel policies and procedures, quality assurance, and outcome evaluation can be addressed through the use of consultants, distance learning, study groups, sharing of critical articles, and Internet access. The Joint Commission on Accreditation of Healthcare Organizations emphasizes this aspect of service delivery and has published helpful manuals, updates, and supporting documents for this purpose.

■ CONSULTATION TO COMMUNITY AGENCIES

Principles of the Consultative Process

Consultation to community agencies is done within a distinctive structure with different processes and expectations than for the work of staff members directly employed by or directing the agency. The levels in which the consultant can practice are analogous to those of the permanent staff—that is, over the entire range of the agency's organization. Consultants are not legally responsible for the actions of agency staff, for implementation of policy decisions, or for employee-related decisions, because they serve as neither a supervisor nor a supervisee. Confidentiality is unidirectional—that is, the consultant is expected not to share information derived from the consultee (the person in the agency receiving consultation) without a prior understanding of how the information will be used; consultees may share the consultation-derived information in any manner they wish. Consultants' authority derives from their specialized expertise in the area in which the agency seeks assistance; the authority of the consultees, regardless of their position within the agency, is based on their knowledge of the agency and its population, rules and regulations, and the culture within which they are employed. Consultants bring their expertise to the agency and contract to provide a service that allows a unique relationship between equals in governing their interaction.

The consultant's role is often blurred. Several models exist for providing consultation to agencies (Altrocchi 1972; Caplan 1970; Fritz et al. 1993; Schwab-Stone et al. 2002), and there is one for consulting to networks (Goodstein 1983). Grigsby (2002) described the provision of consultation to several types of community agencies and entities. The manner in which the consultant is to function and the features of the agency are important considerations. With the development of MCOs and managed systems of care (Pumariega and Winters 2003), "decategorization" of funding sources and blending of funds, a further shift in consultation focus from individual agencies to systems of care can be expected. Consultants are expected to serve as advocates for multiple constituencies; to develop an understanding of the agency and the relationship between its internal and external environment; and then, depending on the contract, to assist the agency in determining its directions, development, and operations. The consultant suggests policy development and its implementation, formulates impressions, helps define options and areas requiring better definition, and develops recommendations at the agency's request.

Several practical issues and ethical dilemmas occur in the consultative process. Lippit (1983) and Altrocchi (1972) got to the core of the consultative process. Before engaging in the consultative process, the consultant should consider several tasks:

- Clarifying values held by the consultant
- Developing skills to use those values in the process
- Learning how to evaluate the consultative work performed

The administrator or consultee may have a similar list, but the manner in which the resultant analysis is employed does differ. At different levels, the consultant may even be simultaneously trusted and mistrusted. Consultation phases have been defined in several ways. Lippit's (1983) definition may prove useful:

- Making initial contact and entry
- Formulating a contract and establishing a working relationship
- Identifying the problem and a diagnosis
- Setting goals and planning for them
- Converting plans into action
- Completing the contract and addressing continuity and support

The reader is encouraged to review the papers by Lippit (1983) and Altrocchi (1972) for more detail and for concrete, well-illustrated examples.

Phases in the Consultative Process

First Contact and Entry Into the Agency

You are contacted by a supervisor at a residential treatment center. She has earned your respect after collaborating with you in treating hyperactive, depressed, and assaultive children. She asks you to come to the center on a regular basis and consult with a group of supervisors who informally meet there weekly to improve their skills and support each other. They are willing to pay about two-thirds of your normal rate. You are thinking about adding consultation to your practice and are pleased with the request.

The following issues require immediate consideration: 1) Why is the request being made now? 2) Who is the consultee? 3) What is the role of the residential program in this process? 4) How will this consultation be viewed by the center administrators? 5) What are the expectations, and how realistic are they? 6) What possible conflicts of interest exist?

A preliminary response could include agreeing to attend an informal meeting if it is approved by the agency's executive director or designee. Such approval would constitute a mandate to continue the process. It should be clarified whether a member of the administration will also be attending the initial meetings. Once permission for involvement with supervisory staff has been granted, the potential consultative relationship can be framed by the questions raised and the information provided. (It is important to remember that the overt question presented in this initial phase is rarely the actual or covert reason for the consultation request.) It is helpful to learn about the supervisors' expectations for the consultation, their conceptions about the consultative process, and (if germane) their earlier experiences with consultants. Models of consultation should be reviewed regarding the anticipated focus or aim of the consultation and its content (described below in this section). It is important to determine whether the supervisors simply wish to get in-service training from an experienced mental health professional who works regularly with disturbed youngsters or whether they wish to work on issues related to being as effective as can reasonably be expected.

In proceeding, the consultant needs to consider potential consultative directions to explore. They fall within the traditional four types described by Caplan (1970):

- Client-centered case consultation (focus is on the individual case at hand)
- Consultee-centered case consultation (focus is on upgrading the consultee for future situations)
- Program-centered consultation (focus is on the program)
- Consultee-centered administrative consultation (focus is on the chief administrator)

Client-centered and consultee-centered case consultations have considerable overlap. For this particular situation, both approaches for the consultees to select can be laid out in a nonthreatening manner. Activities might include the following:

- Sharing knowledge about human development, management of deviant behavior, work with families, collaboration with physicians who prescribe medication, and referrals for assessment or disposition
- Sharing knowledge and assisting with skills development to manage various situations the consultees are likely to face

- Assisting with the planning of new projects or programs, staff development, and training
- Assisting with treatment planning for center residents or their families who have not responded to treatment as expected
- Managing responses of the frontline staff to the residents and their problems

The negative aspects (e.g., being scrutinized, criticized, and evaluated) of the consultation request may be addressed to demonstrate empathy for the meaning of seeking help and opening up the agency for assessment and change.

This first phase sets the stage for the development of a contract and an understanding about working together. The consultant sharing his or her experience in areas of the consultee's concerns can provide impressions about how well the consultant's skills and experiences match the consultee's needs and can also help shape the contract to be negotiated. The consultant may ask to tour the center, meet with supervisors and direct-line staff, visit program components, and attend staff or administrative meetings—all with authorization from the director. It is helpful for the consultant to voice an expectation of learning from the consultation as well as providing the agency and its staff with expertise. Once the consultant understands what the consultees desire from the consultation, and they have a sense of the consultant's style, level of experience, and skill, it is time to enter the next phase of consultation.

Contract Formulation and Developing the Consultative Relationship

This phase takes place after the consultant and the agency have had an opportunity to consider the desirability of continuing with the process, fees for the consultation, issues related to confidentiality, the type of consultation that will be employed, responsibilities of the consultant agency and consultee, the frequency of meetings, the duration of the relationship (i.e., when to end or reevaluate the consultation), and the need to get permission to change the focus of the consultation or to discuss specific children if that is intended. A major pitfall in client-centered case consultation is the attempt by consultees to transfer responsibility to the consultant. This facet and issues related to ownership of consultation data and the handling of confidentiality need to be well defined. Failure to do so can later cause numerous difficulties and can disrupt the consultation. Expectations that the consultants will share impressions with supervisors and administrators about individual or group-member consultees can become stumbling blocks in the consultative process. Questions about how the consultant's impressions or judgments will be used and concerns that the administrator will demand to know who is not functioning well or is problematic are inevitable. Emphatically dealing with these issues early and insisting that rules of confidentiality hold should spare both the consultant and consultee multiple future problems. Depending on the situation, it is usually prudent to leave the consultative focus as open as feasible to allow for potential changes in emphasis as the consultant learns more about the agency and its dynamics. The consultant also should make clear that answers to questions and solutions to problems are expected to come from the consultees through their answers to the questions raised by the consultant from insights developed in the consultative process. The voluntary nature of the consultees' participation must be emphasized, and agreement needs to be reached about the focus and approach of the consultation.

A major concern is the propensity for consultees to ask the consultant to serve in direct-service capacities (e.g., functioning as a supervisor, teacher, or psychotherapist or as the professional to certify treatment for payers such as Medicaid and MCOs). This request most often occurs with professionals who have state licenses and can perform those particular functions. The consultative relationship must drastically change if this kind of shift occurs. The consultant then assumes direct responsibility for the agency's residents, clients, or patients. Supervision, legal liability, and other responsibilities must then be accepted by the consultant. Such developments can be managed if the consultant is aware of the ramifications (e.g., shifting relationships with other staff members). Once the contract is accepted, relationships between the consultant, the agency, and its staff begin to develop. How this phase is handled greatly influences the conduct of the consultation.

The consultation and its ultimate impact can be affected by the attitude and techniques of consultants (Eisdorfer and Batton 1972). The attitudes and techniques of consultants range widely: some consultants dissect agencies to apply a specific theory; others believe that therapy is the solution to all problems; some imagine themselves to be all-knowing or consistently play devil's advocate in all situations; and still others are able to relate well to all. The consultant must be alert to the occurrence of these stereotypical traits, particularly during the earliest stages of the relationship, when these traits are most likely to emerge. The professional style (adjusting to consultee and agency needs within professional boundaries set by the consultation) is associated with the fewest negative connotations. The professional continues to develop an understanding of the agency and its issues as the consultative process proceeds, accepts the consultees as fellow professionals, and assists them in developing an understanding of their situation and finding solutions to their problems.

Problem Identification and Diagnosis

Unless the consultation request is greatly delimited (e.g., a series of lectures or seminars), problem identification and diagnosis is the most difficult phase of the consultative process, because the consultant must set the boundaries of the problem and consider sources of resistance to dealing with it. For example, the consultant should assess the consequences of his or her involvement within the system, including the development of fears, anxieties, and ambivalence about change within the agency or network. Issues related to confidentiality and ownership of data usually arise at this phase and must be addressed. Openness about wanting to understand the system and how it functions can help the consultant to be effective. Recognizing resistance and supporting it to some extent can be useful in allaying undue anxiety. To avoid some of the traps inherent in the consultative situation, it is often necessary to restate that the consultation is to the entire agency. Agreeing to lay out a course of action as soon as feasible is another necessity. It is also essential to have an explicit definition of which information that is shared during the consultation will not be divulged. However, it is advisable to include a proviso whereby the consultant may ask permission to use the information at a later time if it is deemed appropriate and necessary. Recommendations can be made and questions raised without the need for direct revelation of the material shared within the consultative relationship.

This phase and the next, sometimes classified as beginning or warming-up stages, concern both nurturing the relationship and addressing the problem. To be most effective, the consultant should assist the consultee to define the problem and consider alternative solutions while resisting several temptations (e.g., determining the nature of the problem and its solutions without obtaining input from the consultee, or forcing the consultant's own values and goals on alternative choices).

Goal Setting, Planning, and Converting Plans Into Action

The tasks in this phase involve searching for alternative, acceptable actions. The results of these tasks should help the consultees select appropriate courses of action. The consultant needs to have a clear understanding of who has the responsibility and the authority to make decisions. Methods to evaluate agency outcomes must be built into any planned or implemented interventions. By agreeing on the means of evaluating policy changes, the consultant is assisting the consultees to consider various outcomes, both positive and negative. The consultant must be prepared to accept the consultees' right to select and implement courses of action that seem ineffective or ill-advised. If a course of action is likely to fail, the consultant's task is to convey his or her questions and to help develop strategies that can minimize or reverse the damage.

Contract Completion: Termination

Letting go, whether from a therapeutic or a consultative relationship, is difficult. Termination matters must be considered in a measured and deliberate fashion. Criteria for completion should be developed early in the consultation and the process monitored. Relationships become strained when the consultant believes that more is better and the agency does not; this situation calls for maturity and a dose of trust to clarify matters and to allow differences in perception to be settled. Determining how and when it is ethical and appropriate for the consultant to employ insights gained from the consultation to advocate for children and adolescents in the agency and other contexts is sometimes problematic. Reviewing the data collected, issues remaining for the agency, and progress achieved generally suffices for the exit review. The success of the consultation may be measured in various ways, but only longitudinal evaluation can provide definitive answers. Means for such evaluation should be developed early in the consultation and should be in place for longitudinal data collection. Examples of such measures are provided in the chapters that follow. Setting a date to review the data allows for closure and provides an opportunity to conduct quality assurance and performance improvement and to decide whether to broaden or continue the consultative relationship. Consultation to community agencies is a simple process with several very complex interactions that the mental health consultant must be alert for and willing to address. Working with HSAs provides community mental health professionals—especially in the consultative process—the opportunity to multiply their talents, skills, and efforts for the benefit of those in the community who are most in need of their assistance.

▌ CONCLUSIONS

As HSAs confront the current political and fiscal landscape, increases in the employment of professionals and others with mental health credentials can be expected. Practice and consultation in community settings as a CMHW is challenging and rewarding. The responsibility to ensure equitable delivery of quality services to a very needy population can seem daunting. This chapter outlines factors for consideration in assessing the environment, the tasks such effort entails, and the role of the consultant. Subsequent chapters cover the concepts discussed here in greater depth and specificity regarding agencies or activities that are likely venues for CMHW practice and consultation.

▌ REFERENCES

Altrocchi J: Mental health consultation, in Handbook of Community Mental Health. Edited by Golann SE, Eisdorfer C. New York, Appleton-Century-Crofts, 1972, pp 477–508
Caplan G: Theory and Practice of Mental Health Consultation. New York, Basic Books, 1970

Eisdorfer C, Batton L: The mental health consultant as seen by his consultees. Community Ment Health J 8:171–177, 1972

Fritz GK, Mattison RE, Nurcombe B, et al: Child and Adolescent Mental Health Consultation in Hospitals, Schools, and Courts. Washington, DC, American Psychiatric Press, 1993

Goodstein LD: Consultation to human service networks, in The Mental Health Consultation Field. Edited by Cooper S, Hodges WF. New York, Human Sciences Press, 1983, pp 267–287

Grigsby RK: Consultation with foster care homes, group homes, youth shelters, domestic violence shelters, and big brothers/big sisters programs, in Child and Adolescent Psychiatry: A Comprehensive Textbook, 3rd Edition. Edited by Lewis M. Philadelphia, PA, Lippincott Williams & Wilkins, 2002, pp 1393–1398

Individuals With Disabilities Act, Pub. L. No. 101-476

Lippit R: Ethical issues and criteria in intervention decisions, in The Mental Health Consultation Field. Edited by Cooper S, Hodges WF. New York, Human Sciences Press, 1983, pp 139–151

Pumariega AJ, Winters NC (eds): The Handbook of Child and Adolescent Systems of Care: The New Community Psychiatry. San Francisco, CA, Wiley, 2003

Schwab-Stone ME, Henrich C, Armbruster P: School consultation, in Child and Adolescent Psychiatry: A Comprehensive Textbook, 3rd Edition. Edited by Lewis M. Philadelphia, PA, Lippincott Williams & Wilkins, 2002, pp 1361–1370

Weisbord MR: Organizational Diagnosis: A Workbook of Theory and Practice. Reading, MA, Addison-Wesley, 1978

2 PUBLIC-SECTOR DYNAMICS FOR CHILD MENTAL HEALTH

Theodore Fallon, M.D., M.P.H.

Judith Dogin, M.D.

The exponential growth of children's mental health services since World War II has created the need to understand and guide delivery of these services. Historically, these services were conceptualized as being either in the private sector or in the public sector. The public sector comprised government-funded community mental health and child guidance centers providing care for a population of children and families who were unable to pay for care themselves. Public funds were limited and had to provide for an entire population defined by low income.

The health care system in the United States has recently become more complex. Many states have channeled government funds, particularly Title XIX (Medicaid), to privately operated managed care systems. Conversely, private health care organizations have engaged large numbers of practitioners to care for populations of patients who are capitated by virtue of their place of employment. The distinction between public and private has become blurred. But if *public sector* is defined as a population of people clustered together for the purpose of pooling funds for health care, then this term has a much broader applicability. It refers to situations in which a defined population is underwritten by a third-party payer. This third party could be a health maintenance organization (HMO), a managed care organization, a traditional health insurance company, or a government-funded program. Three elements characterize the public sector:

1. The *population* that defines the sector. (For Medicaid, this population would be low-income families; for an HMO, it would be all members of the HMO. All members of the population, however, do not need care.)
2. The *individuals* within the population who need care: patients.
3. The *resources* available to the population. (In the case of a publicly funded child guidance clinic, the resources would be the funds provided to the clinic. In the case of an HMO, the resources would be the pool of money available to fund the care.)

The term *dynamics* alludes to nonstatic forces between elements. *Public-sector dynamics* therefore refers to the tripartite relationship and interactions among three elements: the population as a whole, the individual patients, and the health care resources available. In this dynamic interchange, understanding and monitoring these elements and the relationships among them is critical to a balanced mental health system that tends to the needs of each individual—as well as to the larger population—in a way that maximizes the available resources. These relationships are measured by examining *efficiency*, the degree to which resources are used judiciously; and *effectiveness*, the extent to which morbidity and mortality can be prevented. In this way, prevention becomes an important element of public-sector dynamics.

Mental health prevention can be defined in three ways:

1. *Primary prevention* comprises activities by which psychopathology is avoided throughout the entire population.
2. *Secondary prevention* comprises treatments that reverse psychopathology after it has been manifested (a cure).
3. *Tertiary prevention* comprises treatments that minimize or prevent damage from psychopathology, even though the psychopathology cannot be cured.

There is natural tension among the three different public-sector elements (population needs, individual patient needs, and available resources). The concept of prevention particularly highlights this tension when one considers the efficiency and effectiveness of primary prevention versus secondary and tertiary prevention. How much of the available community resources should go to each type of prevention?

But even within a particular level of prevention, many issues must be considered when thinking about effective and efficient use of resources. Consider the comparison of an anorexic girl in a suburban child guidance clinic versus an angry, gun-toting youth in an urban mental health clinic. The girl may threaten her own life, whereas the urban youth threatens the lives of others. Each setting has different resource availability, different populations, and different cultural and environmental demands. Balancing individual patients' needs, the community's needs, and the available resources is common sense, but this balance is easily overlooked and not always easy to do; information to permit understanding these dynamics must be sought out and integrated. This chapter provides a step-by-step guide on how to consider public-sector dynamics by 1) providing a conceptual framework; 2) exploring ways this framework can lead to an assessment of the system, which includes assessing the three public-sector elements and their interactions; and 3) offering goals that can help guide in designing, constructing, administering, and working to create a balanced mental health system of care.

▌ A CONCEPTUAL FRAMEWORK

In the United States before World War II, patient care operated mostly in a free-market system with little consideration for the needs of the entire population. A patient wanted services, and a practitioner offered them. This transaction took place only between the practitioner and the patient; because all patients paid their practitioners directly, the clinicians' sole responsibility and allegiance were to the patients. The good of the community did not usually enter into consideration. There were publicly funded services and considerations for public and community health, but the general practice of caring for patients took place in the private sector between patient and practitioner.

After World War II, third parties gradually became involved in medical care in the form of health insurance, government programs (e.g., Medicaid, Medicare, disability, worker's compensation, and community health and mental health clinics), and HMOs—and the public sector was born. Patients were no longer limited by their own personal resources in obtaining health care, and practitioners were no longer restricted in providing care and using resources for their patients. A seemingly bottomless wellspring of resources could be dipped into whenever anyone was ill. Initially, this arrangement seemed utopian; however, conflict inevitably arose with the recognition that the wellspring was not bottomless. A demand to balance competing interests ensued. In child mental health, recognition of the conflict has come only gradually. There seem to be two complex reasons for this:

1. Although a considerable amount of knowledge abounds on what is needed to provide optimally for the psychological development of chil-

dren, it has been difficult to use this knowledge to design and carry out effective, efficient treatments. The difficulty pertains to a complex and massive knowledge in the field that can only be contained by dozens of disciplines, and many agencies and organizations have not been able to coordinate efforts.

2. With an in-depth understanding of the complexities of child development, it is possible to begin to see the nuances of its deviations—and the enormous unmet needs in large segments of the population. Because the implications of this enormous unmet need are overwhelming for society, most people in the general public (including policy makers and taxpayers) are reluctant to acknowledge these needs.

As a result, community mental health programs either have frighteningly few resources for children or include inadvertent loopholes that allow unlimited access to resources, resulting in staggering budgets. It is rare (if not unheard of) to find rational resource allocation in a children's mental health program that is driven by an understanding of child development. Such a rational approach requires knowledge of the needs of individual patients, knowledge of the needs of the overall population, and knowledge of the available resources.

The field of public mental health demonstrates some experience in this rational approach. Community mental health centers (CMHCs), initially funded during the Kennedy administration, have always dealt with a fixed pool of resources. But incentives toward developing more effective, efficient treatments were lacking in these early systems of care. Managed care organizations have recently attempted to introduce potential competition and risk, but the motivation of for-profit agencies is to minimize cost, not to optimize the long-term psychological development of children. As the face of health care delivery changes, the public sector will likely pervade an even larger segment of mental health care than it has previously. If the voices of individuals and the general population are included in this process, at least there will be an ever-present pressure to balance the population's needs, individual patients' needs, and available resources.

To construct a mental health system that can rationally balance the three elements, there must be clinical and administrative personnel within the system who have the following attributes:

- Ability to assess the three elements within the system of care (individual patient needs, community needs, and resource availability)
- Knowledge of how to balance the competing interests
- Power to allocate resources appropriately

█ ASSESSMENT

An assessment of the entire system of care is comparable in utility to the clinical diagnostic evaluation. For example, in a system with more patients to treat than resources available, an assessment of the three elements is imperative. Only when there is a clear understanding of the scope and magnitude of the needs can there be dialogue and thinking leading to a solution that balances the needs of individual patients with the needs and resources of the community. Other political, social, fiscal, and organizational forces also will demand consideration.

Individual Patient Needs

The assessment and monitoring of each element of care have traditionally been done in different fields. Mental health clinicians have routinely performed assessments of individual patients, a skill that requires training and experience. Because a great deal has been written about assessment and it is covered elsewhere in this book, the topic is not covered here. Important to acknowledge, however, is that the results of patient assessment and treatment recommendations will vary considerably between clinicians. Although this variability would be a problem if the goal were data collection for research or quality control of a production line, in this context it can be seen as lending richness to the field and allowing clinical work to evolve. Another important aspect of patient assessment is its ongoing nature. The continual monitoring of individual patients, which of course is an integral part of any good treatment, allows the clinician to make progressively closer approximations to an individual's true need and protects against incorrect assessments.

Community Needs

To balance the particular needs of any individual against the overall need of the community, the community's needs must be assessed. Epidemiology, the study of populations, is useful here. Psychiatric epidemiological instruments and techniques have developed considerably since the 1960s, but epidemiological data are limited in the picture they can provide. Without individual cases, epidemiological information by itself can provide only circumstantial information. Epidemiological data are distant from patients, evincing directions and trends but not actual individual circumstances, like a road map that provides directions but does not illuminate detailed features of the land itself. In addition, the science and technology of psychiatric epidemiology are still in the process of being developed, particularly with regard to children and families. The process of identifying community needs has three steps:

1. Identifying the target population
2. Assessing needs
3. Identifying the types of needed services

Defining the Target Population

The first task in a population assessment is to identify the community to be served—or, in epidemiological terms, to define the target population (usually defined by the total number of potential patients). For a geographical region such as a catchment area, the target population is the entire population within the geographical bounds. For an HMO, the target population is the subscribers. For a single CMHC, the definition of the target population is usually more complex: it must include consideration of the mandate of the agency, funding sources, and the availability of other providers.

Most CMHCs cover a segment of a geographical population. For example, a clinic might be funded by the state child protective agency. Such funding would then mandate that the clinic serve the families and children within the child protective population. Private practice or other mental health agencies may cover other segments of the population. The child protective agency may also fund other clinics in the area, which would necessitate coordination with these other clinics in defining the target population. Lack of coordination among agencies is sometimes the greatest impediment to defining the target population. This coordination might be carried out by the funding agencies, governmental agencies, the service providers themselves, or some combination.

For a geographically based population, conducting house-to-house surveys of the number of children to delineate the target population may provide the most accurate data; however, U.S. Census data, which are gathered every 10 years, makes this sort of surveying unnecessary. These data can be obtained from the U.S. Census Bureau (customer service in Washington, D.C., 301-763-4100 or through the Internet at http://www.census.gov). A neighborhood statistics program connected with regional statistics bureaus around the country can assist in processing these data. These programs are usually based within state agencies.

The publicly funded West Haven Community Mental Health Center is in a working-class town of 54,000 people (according to U.S. Census data). Like two other local CMHCs, West Haven Community Mental Health Center is mandated to provide mental health services to children and families who cannot obtain these services from other sources. Private practitioners are available to see children and families with private insurance, and these practitioners rarely see patients who do not have private insurance. The target population is partly defined by indigent children on welfare and those without insurance. This population, however, is served by the three local public CMHCs. As an estimate of the target population, the U.S. Census data for 2000 indicate that 12,000 children reside in the town of West Haven and about 1,000 of them live in households with income below the poverty level. If children living in households with income less than $30,000 are included to estimate the number of children without adequate insurance, this adds another 5,000 children to the total, for a target population of approximately 6,000 children served by the three CMHCs in the area.

For planning and resource distribution purposes, it is important to define how these clinics share the target population, although political agendas interfere with this process. In this particular example, resource distribution is determined by the funding agency that allocates funding among the three CMHCs. Missing from this process is a mechanism that links funding with responsibility for care of a segment of the population. Historically, this mechanism was achieved by establishing catchment areas, although this practice has recently fallen into disfavor.

Assessing Needs

Once the target population is identified, it is then useful for planning purposes to estimate the number of individuals within this target population who will need care. This process, known as a *needs assessment,* allows identification of the subpopulations that actually require care.

Of the many ways to assess the needs of a community, some are more precise and some are more expedient. The most precise is the direct epidemiological assessment of the target population. For example, all subscribers to an HMO or a managed care entity might be sent a mental health screening questionnaire. Similarly, a written questionnaire might be sent to all the patients of certain pediatricians if the target population is contained within certain identified pediatric practices (Jellinek and associates have designed such an instrument, available at http://www.massgeneral.org/allpsych/PediatricSymptomChecklist/psc_home.htm). This type of assessment requires distribution of the questionnaires or even door-to-door surveys, then data entry and analysis, all of which can be quite expensive. More practical and expedient methods of assessing community needs include the following:

• Use of data that have already been gathered
• Surveys of referral sources
• Use of estimates found in the existing literature

Considerable information that can be useful in assessing the community is often already available, although some work might be necessary to get the data into a usable form. Community indicators for mental health services for children might include data on truancy; delinquency; physical health problems; child protective service referrals; and service use obtained through schools, law enforcement agencies, public health departments, and mental health clinics themselves. These data, along with census data, provide rough estimates of the numbers of children and families in need of mental health care.

Surveying referral sources can also provide estimates of need. For example, if pediatricians are a major source of referrals, then asking all or a sample of pediatricians how many of their patients might benefit from mental health care may provide sufficient information. Referrals through public services (child protective systems, juvenile justice departments, the courts, law enforcement agencies, the schools, and even the police) are particularly important in the public sector. Many of these public agencies already identify and track high-risk children and families.

Unless an agency has a particular mandate to see referrals from only one source, it will be necessary to canvass a number of referral sources. Each referral source, of course, will have its own type of patient. For example, the juvenile justice system by definition identifies delinquents but will usually refer patients who need treatment for psychosis, depression, suicidal ideation, and substance use. Schools tend to refer children who engage in disruptive behavior. In fact, most agencies tend to refer children with disruptive behaviors, because the attention-demanding symptoms of such children make their need for services evident to those around them. Children with more internal disorders such as depression or anxiety are more likely to be identified by people in the community who have known them for a prolonged period of time (e.g., parents, clergy, block group leaders, scout leaders, and coaches).

It is also important to keep in mind possible biases that are inherent in data used to estimate needs. For example, when using data from referral agencies, it is important to remember that referring pediatricians, teachers, lawyers, parole officers, and police officers are not trained in mental health diagnosis. A review of the literature suggests that pediatricians are capable of detecting severe mental health problems but are poor at detecting mild and moderate problems (Lavigne et al. 1993).

Using published estimates of the need for mental health treatment can be even more expedient. In the literature, prevalence estimates of psychiatrically disturbed children range from 12% to 25% of the general population, but only 3%–6% of the general population have severe disturbances. On the other hand, estimates of the use of mental health services have historically been about 2% of the general population per year. The segment of the population served can vary considerably depending on local conditions. For example, researchers in the Fort Bragg study found that if exceptional services are offered, up to 8% of the child population will use them (Bickman 1995).

Returning to the example of the West Haven Community Mental Health Center, if one uses the national estimate of 3%–6% of the population being seriously emotionally disturbed and another 5%–10% of the population being less seriously disturbed but still in need of treatment at any one time, then in the target population of 6,000 the potential number of individuals who need treatment is perhaps 180–300, and another 300–600 children might benefit from treatment. The capacity of the West Haven Community Mental Health Center is about 150 youngsters in treatment at any one time, leaving 330–750 children to be seen by the other two clinics. In fact, those clinics together see about 200 West Haven children, leaving 130–550 children with severe disturbances who are not seen at any of the clinics.

Estimates suggest that, nationally, only 20%–40% of children who might benefit from treatment actually receive it. In West Haven, 40%–70% of children who need treatment receive it. These rough calculations suggest that the quantity of mental health care available in the West Haven community is at least comparable if not superior to that found in the rest of the country. At the same time, 30%–60% of West Haven children who need treatment are not receiving it. Therefore, the need for additional service has been demonstrated.

Identifying Types of Needed Services

The purpose of a mental health needs assessment is to identify both a subpopulation in need and the particular types of needs of that subpopulation. This further refinement of the needs assessment can be done by gathering more details using the methods described in the section above. The most expedient (although least complete) of these methods is to assess the population of patients who present themselves for services to the practitioners who see them. Mental health practitioners may be the most sensitive to some of the particular types of needs with which patients and their families present. One could also assess patients as they enter the clinic, using instruments such as the Child and Adolescent Service Intensity Instrument (CASII; available through the American Academy of Child and Adolescent Psychiatry at http://www.aacap.org/clinical/CASII/index.htm). This scale (formerly the Child and Adolescent Level of Care Utilization System; CALOCUS) is particularly useful if resources are available that address a continuum of service-need intensities (e.g., inpatient, residential, intensive outpatient, day treatment, or standard outpatient). However, if one is attempting to understand the types of psychopathology in order to design services, then the Child Behavior Checklist or a related instrument might be more appropriate as an initial intake tool.

Using a combination of practitioner observation, patient surveys, and epidemiological techniques, the West Haven Community Mental Health Center identified a need for parent training. On a routine question to families at intake about whether or not they had ever been involved in child protective services, only 2% answered affirmatively. Cross-referenced patient lists with the local child protective service, however, indicated that more than 50% of these families were either active child protective cases or had been active in the past 2 years. For confidentiality reasons, the clinic was not able to identify specific families, but clinicians became much more sensitive to these issues. By understanding these needs, administrators and clinicians working together designed efficient, effective, and easy-to-use intake, tracking, and discharge procedures that maximized parent training.

Thus, important but unexpected information can be gained in the course of performing a needs assessment.

In another clinic serving a Puerto Rican immigrant population, it was discovered that parents of child patients almost uniformly had less than a fourth-grade education. This information was useful in planning for services and was also helpful to the clinicians in assessing the level of understanding among these parents. Given this information, it was also not surprising to discover that this population had tremendous difficulty negotiating with personnel in most public agencies. The difficulty helped explain the high rate of child protective service referrals and the large number of children in this population who had been removed from their homes. With this information, clinicians worked to be more sensitive to families' informational needs and also worked to help educate the child protective service workers involved with these families.

When adequate information gathering and needs assessment of the population have not been performed, clinicians and administrators may not be aware of significant mental health needs within the target population, especially when these patients do not present themselves for treatment. In many communities, discrete groups of patients in the target population need treatment but are not receiving it. These groups are often identifiable by particular referral sources. Finding these groups requires both exploration within the community and detailed needs assessments as described earlier in this section. Although many of the most seriously disturbed children (e.g., acting-out adolescents) will be identified by multiple agencies, other children are less likely to be identified (e.g., children with depressive or anxiety disorders).

With the information gathered from the population and from more specific assessments, a clearer picture of both community and patient needs comes into view. With this clarity, administrative procedures and clinical services can be designed and targeted. Once new services or procedures have been put in place, reassessment might begin to show the effectiveness of these new additions. This feedback is crucial to guide further refinement of services and procedures. In deciding what reassessments should be performed, it is important to consider the agency's mission as well as the population that is being served and the available resources to support that work.

Administrative procedures and high no-show rates bogged down the West Haven Community Mental Health Center intake procedure while leaving clinicians unproductive. A new solution to this problem was desperately needed. Creating routine intake times at which several new patients could be easily scheduled and making a pool of clinicians available to see these new patients allowed for a 20-fold increase in the clinic's ability to accept new referrals.

If untreated populations are identified, cooperative efforts between administrators and clinicians provide the best opportunity for devising efficient, effective, and easy-to-use administrative procedures. These cooperative efforts usually need to be extended across agencies so that they can address some difficult-to-reach populations. For example, for adolescents within a juvenile justice system to get mental health evaluation and treatment, cooperative agreement between the juvenile probation department and a mental health clinic may be needed. Moreover, identification of previously unidentified populations of children in need of mental health services may offer fertile ground for further collaboration, including funding opportunities and preventive interventions.

Resource Availability

Resources are services that can be brought to bear to assist patients and their families. These resources include clinician service hours, expert consultation, support services, and the like. For any clinic, the resources can usually be enumerated. For services in the broader community, lists are available, usually from federal, state, and local funding agencies. In metropolitan areas, the list can be overwhelming. Managing available resources has been the purview of insurance companies, organizational managers, case managers, health service researchers, and public officials.

Garnering children's mental health resources may happen in a variety of ways, including finding available services, creating resources through political means, redirecting available funds by convincing those with the authority to do so, or cultivating volunteer sources of money or personnel. Political influence also can be extremely important. One can have influence through direct connections with local, state, and federal officials. A recommended approach is calling a legislator's office and making an appointment to discuss concerns. These concerns should be presented from the perspective of the legislator's constituents, using the data that have been gathered and the visiting clinician's professional opinion to justify a given position. Although children's interests are relatively poorly attended to in the political system, politicians and especially the general public are sympathetic and responsive when obvious need and urgency are demonstrated.

Funding

Sometimes local governments and foundations will have special initiatives for children. Both public and private organizations regularly issue requests for proposals soliciting providers of various services. Local and state child protective agencies, juvenile justice systems, schools, police departments, departments of health and mental health, the National Institute of Mental Health, and private foundations are additional funding sources. The federal government and many state and metropolitan areas maintain Web sites advertising these proposals. Individuals, services, and databases can assist in locating national and local funding sources for grant monies. *The Foundation Directory,* published by The Foundation Center in New York (http://fdncenter.org), is one such source, but many others are available on the World Wide Web.

▋ GOALS

The ultimate goals of community mental health services are preventing emotional pain and suffering before it begins (primary prevention), minimizing it after it has begun (secondary prevention), and preventing further deterioration (tertiary prevention). These goals require knowing the at-risk populations in all their forms. If these broad goals are applied to the model presented in this chapter, then the ultimate test of the successful balancing of individual and community needs with available resources will be the effective and efficient use of the available resources in primary, secondary, and tertiary prevention. The measurement of this prevention would involve identifying, assessing, and following up on fairly large segments of the population over their lifetimes to see the effects of any efforts.

Methods to identify at-risk populations are still in the early stages of development. Much is yet to be understood about the effects of therapeutic activities on at-risk populations. The actual measurement of progress is fraught with difficulties because there are few existing standardized outcome measures for the mental health, well-being, and psychological development of individuals, let alone of communities. Available measures may not be responsive to the types of intervention that are currently provided. Some community indicators (e.g., crime statistics, incidence of child welfare referrals, or adolescent pregnancy and high school dropout rates) may reflect changes, although they monitor the negative side of mental health. Evaluation efforts require persistence; measuring progress could possibly take years or even generations. If child mental health is to be responsive to the community as well as to the individual, then better outcome measures must be developed.

Further Refinement of the Dynamic Model: Allocation of Resources

The dearth of outcome measures means that an interim mechanism is needed to facilitate the balancing of individual patient needs, population needs, and available resources. Although various methods have been (and are being) tried for allocating these resources (e.g., micromanaged managed care), it is important to remember the implications of Milgram's studies in the late 1960s: the further removed a decision maker is from those affected by his or her decisions, the more willing that decision maker is to inflict pain (Milgram 1968). Perhaps the best person to weigh individual and community interests is a well-informed clinician who is closest to the individual and the community being served. Because clinicians are primarily trained in assessing individual needs, it then becomes imperative that practitioners be trained to know the community and available resources and to understand the implications of balancing this equation. Operationally, this means that for each case, the clinician should consider the needs and desires of the child and family, the community's needs and desires, and the resources available to address those needs. In some cases, it may mean that the clinician must acknowledge having neither the knowledge nor the resources to address these problems to the desired extent. The clinician's clear conflict of interest in serving the patient but holding the community's interests in mind is precisely why the clinician is the best person to make decisions regarding available resources. The clinician must recognize the limits of his or her ability to help in making critical decisions about available resources. Failure to do so is tantamount to abdicating control of important resources. Failure to represent all interests in the arbitrating process results in opposition by interests that are not represented and may be the primary reason why micromanaged managed care has been able to develop. In the past, well-trained clinicians were able to garner the public trust. Clinicians of the twenty-first century will be able to maintain this trust only if they are able to represent and have the endorsement of most if not all aspects of the increasingly complex health system and community. In this formula, an understanding not only of the systems of care but also of all the stakeholders involved in the care is necessary.

Clinicians who can well represent the community's desires and needs must be able to track these, make decisions, and justify these decisions regarding community interests. Obtaining input from community boards representing various community factions is one way to get input regarding community desires and needs. Good assessments can help guide the process and can lend political and rhetorical weight. An understanding of the role of the care provider and the clinic within the larger system of care is also important. The identification of this role within a larger system is determined by one's mission and by the community's needs. Alliance and coordination with other agencies that serve children can establish a critical resource for obtaining information and assistance in the delivery of services to the most difficult-to-treat children who require the involvement of multiple agencies. Such alliances can also evolve into lobbying efforts to gain more resources for the entire field.

> After cataloging the child service agencies in the community, the West Haven Community Mental Health Center joined with the public school district, child protective services, the department of public health, and several other agencies to create a community network consisting of child-serving agencies and consumers. Representatives of this network met regularly to discuss the needs of individual patients and of the community. This network served the triple functions of 1) addressing families and children who needed the involvement of multiple agencies; 2) providing a functional assessment of the community's resources, needs, and desires; and 3) coordinating the activities of these agencies within the community. Through the network's coordinated political power, the attention of the town and state governments was drawn to children's needs, and funds were obtained for new programs in juvenile justice.

■ CONCLUSIONS

Because the distinction between public and private sectors of the mental health field are being blurred, the need to comprehend the complex dynamics of the public sector has gained paramount importance. In this chapter, we have provided the reader with concepts and tools to understand and help shape the allocation of scarce resources within the public mental health system.

■ REFERENCES

Bickman L: Evaluating Managed Mental Health Services: The Fort Bragg Experiment. New York, Plenum Press, 1995

Lavigne JV, Binns HJ, Christoffel KK, et al: Behavioral and emotional problems among preschool children in pediatric primary care: prevalence and pediatricians recognition. Pediatrics 91:649–655, 1993

Milgram S: Some conditions of obedience and disobedience to authority. Int J Psychiatry. 4:259–276, 1968

3 LEGAL ISSUES

Richard J. Lawlor, Ph.D., J.D.

Clinicians working with children face additional legal issues regarding evaluation and treatment than do clinicians working with adults. In this chapter, I present general legal principles and emphasize specific areas of concern for the reader working with children and their families. Practitioners in the United States must look first to their own unique state laws, because state laws often differ significantly on these various issues. Clinicians must be aware of the laws within their jurisdiction. These are usually found in the annotated code dealing with the statutory law and in the case law that interprets the statutes in a particular jurisdiction. One can think of *statutory law* enacted by the legislature as a skeleton or framework and of *case law* that interprets a particular statute as skin that fills out and completes the understanding of that law. An *annotated code* presents information by each code section and also refers readers to any cases interpreting that particular section of the law.

Clinicians should be aware that the United States has four sources of law. A full understanding of the law would require researching all four areas to seek any relevant material dealing with the clinician's particular question: federal and state constitutions, federal and state statutory law, federal and state case law, and administrative law at both the federal and the state level. Answers to questions that practicing clinicians have are usually found in state statutory and case law. But certain issues (e.g., federal regulations dealing with treatment of alcohol and drug abuse) are also covered in federal statutory and case law. Other areas (e.g., issues of clinician scope of practice and licensure or certification) are covered in state statutory, case, and perhaps administrative law. When particular problems arise, community mental health workers should always consult with either their own attorney or the attorney for the agency where they work. As a general rule, the law will apply uniformly to clinicians whether they are working in the community, in an agency or institution, or in private practice.

▌ IMPORTANT GENERAL AREAS OF LAW FOR CLINICIANS

Scope of Practice

Clinicians must be aware of the licensure or certification law dealing with their particular profession and must keep abreast of changes in those laws. A practical way of considering licensure or certification is to view the treatment of any human condition as the practice of medicine. Nonphysicians cannot legally treat any human condition. Exceptions to this general rule are made for the various certified and licensed professions: social work, psychology, nursing, marriage and family counseling, and the like. The certification or licensure laws of these various professions can legitimately be conceived of as state permission to carry out a portion of what can be viewed as the practice of medicine. The certification or licensure laws generally define the scope of practice for a particular profession, that is, what a clinician may or may not do. Of particular importance is what the state certification or licensure law says about the diagnosis and treatment of mental disorders. Many states reserve diagnosis and treatment to the practice of psychiatrists (physicians), and any evaluation procedures or treatment carried out by other mental health professionals must be done under the supervision of a licensed physician. In other states, one or more of the mental health professions may have within their scope of practice the right to both diagnose and treat mental disorders independently. Such issues can be important, particularly in small and rural communities where a nonphysician clinician may be practicing in relative isolation, having contact with a psychiatrist only at certain intervals. If supervision is required, the clinician must be aware of and sensitive to these obligations. This issue is becoming increasingly important with the emphasis by many managed care organizations (MCOs) on using less-than-doctoral–level clinicians—including in some instances baccalaureate-level clinicians—to provide services. Clinicians who exceed the scope of their practice place themselves at serious legal risk. Many state statutes provide for disciplinary action in those instances. MCOs cannot grant permission for clinicians to practice beyond the scope of their practice. Clinicians should work out the appropriate supervisory arrangements as needed.

Managed Care Issues

Clinicians are aware that the managed care environment frequently makes both initial evaluation and treatment more difficult and restrictive, but clinicians often do not adequately understand that managed care is a form of insurance. Bewildering arrays of managed care currently exist across states. The forms of managed care range from health maintenance organizations (HMOs) to preferred provider organizations, limited HMOs, individual practice associations, and MCOs. Generally, these various forms function to move from a fee-based service, which employs retroactive or retrospective utilization review, to procedures providing for prospective utilization review of mental health care procedures. The particular types of organizations available within the clinician's jurisdiction are detailed in the insurance section of the statutory code. Some states have many variants of these organizations and other states have few, but the variety of different forms of managed care is increasing.

A clinician should also learn if his or her state law has "any willing provider" clauses, which require that insurance companies keep the panels for these organizations open to any clinician who meets their qualifications. Even more important is the emerging trend of courts to interpret managed care contracts. Legal or ethical considerations may arise in situations where an MCO either denies or severely limits authorization for evaluation or treatment. A series of California court cases (*Wickline v. California* 1986; *Wilson v. Blue Cross of Southern California* 1990) suggest that if the clinician's judgment indicates that treatment or further treatment is needed, the patient must either receive that treatment or be transferred to another provider. The clinician cannot abandon the patient or refuse to provide treatment just because the insurer denies treatment. These cases also indicate that unjustified intrusion by an MCO in its utilization review procedures exposes it to liability if the patient is harmed as a result of these procedures. However, another finding in these cases is that clinicians *must* utilize all available appeal procedures or be personally held liable for any harm that may come to the patient from not receiving needed treatment. Several state legislatures have been working on legislative attempts to hold MCOs liable in cases of malpractice, and clinicians need to consult local laws to ascertain the extent to which MCOs are liable to be sued in these cases. Currently, the ability to directly sue a managed care company is severely limited.

Malpractice Issues

At one time, suits against mental health practitioners were relatively rare, and judgments against them even rarer. There has recently been a significant increase in the number of suits filed against mental health professionals, with most of them falling into the malpractice area of tort law (i.e., negligent or intentional wrongs done by one person to another person and for which the party doing the wrong may be held liable). For a determination of malpractice, the mental health professional must have assumed a professional relationship with the other party that would impose a duty of care. There must also be evidence that the duty of care was breached and that some harm occurred to that party that was caused by the breach of the duty. The elements of malpractice therefore are establishment of a duty, a finding of breach of that duty, establishment that harm occurred, and proof that the harm was caused by the actions or omissions involved in the breach of the duty. Virtually all torts for which suits are brought involve negligent wrongs or harms. Intentional torts would most likely involve assault and battery (e.g., forced use of medication or improper use of restraints), false imprisonment (e.g., failure to follow procedures for proper commitment), sexual misconduct with patients, and perhaps abandonment of a patient. More likely areas for suits involve claims of negligence against a mental health practitioner, and the most significant ones involve breaches of confidentiality for privileged communication, failure to warn third parties of dangerous threats or actions on the part of a patient, improper diagnosis, failure to obtain informed consent, negligent release of patients, and negligent supervision of mental health practitioners working under another clinician. Mental health practitioners should be certain that they are covered by either their own personal professional liability insurance or a policy of their agency.

The distinction between a malpractice action that is brought under a theory of negligence and one brought under a theory of intentional wrongdoing is important for clinicians. Under most state laws, plaintiffs (the patient or family) in a negligence-based lawsuit are allowed to recover actual (compensatory) damages only and cannot recover punitive damages. Under a malpractice action based on an intentional tort, the patient-plaintiff has available the potential to recover punitive damages. Punitive damages, designed to make an example of the offending clinician, can run up to hundreds of times the actual damages sustained by the patient. Besides this chilling effect, most malpractice insurance policies exclude intentional torts and coverage for punitive damages. The malpractice policy covers the expenses of the clinician's defense against a claim of intentional harm, but if the clinician is found to be liable (e.g., in a case involving sexual involvement with a patient), the policy will usually exclude insurance coverage for those damages.

Maintaining Competency

Standards for what is considered competent practice in the mental health arena are constantly evolving. Clinicians must be aware not only of research advances in the field dealing with evolving standards but also of any case law that might impose new standards (e.g., in the 1976 California case of *Landeros v. Flood,* a clinician's behavior in the emergency room was found to be lacking because evidence of child abuse was not reported). Today, most state laws require reporting of any evidence or suspicions of child abuse and neglect. Case law such as that found in *Landeros* can redefine the standard of care.

Clinicians face a wide variety of children's mental health and legal issues. For example, clinicians are involved with children and adolescents whose parents are divorcing and are engaged in custody disputes. Clinicians become involved with families in which allegations of abuse and sexual abuse are made. Clinicians may be involved with minors who are seeking assistance in the areas of abortion, birth control, treatment of sexually transmitted diseases, and the like. Standards of care are emerging in all of these areas, and clinicians who are unaware of either the research literature or the legal literature in these areas function at their own risk.

A classic example of clinicians functioning on clinical intuition when in fact an abundant research base exists is the investigation of child sexual abuse. In every area of the country, there are clinicians who develop reputations for being useful to child protective service authorities by using therapy as a way to get children to talk in cases where there are suspicions of abuse. Clinical lore exists that these children are able to reveal abuse once they have experienced the safety of the therapeutic alliance. No research supports this lore. However, abundant psychological research supports the effects of suggestive interviewing, use of leading questions, repetitive interviewing, and the suggestibility of children's memories. The problems involved with young children who have not developed the capacity to monitor the sources of their information are well documented as one of the major causes of false memories in children induced by inappropriate discussion and questioning, either in therapy or elsewhere. Clinicians unfamiliar with this research literature as well as the problem of source monitoring for children under age 7 operate at their own risk. Numerous lawsuits currently are pending against therapists who have testified that children have been abused and that the therapist can tell from their therapy sessions that this abuse occurred. The research literature does not validate the use of therapy as an investigative technique (Ceci and Bruck 1995; Lawlor 1998).

Risk Assessment

Another area with a constantly changing research base is that of risk assessment and prediction of dangerousness. Well into the 1980s, it was generally taken as a maxim that clinicians could not reliably predict dangerousness. This is still somewhat true today, but now training is available for clinicians to better predict dangerousness or provide a risk assessment more reliably. In fact, clinicians who are familiar with the research about interviewing patients are able to make accurate predictions approximately 60% of the time (Mossman 1994; Otto 1992). Without in-depth knowledge of this research area, however, clinicians are incapable of making these types of assessments. The prediction of dangerousness in children is an extremely difficult area, and at present this type of risk assessment does not have the research base that is available to clinicians working with adults. Until this base is developed, clinicians would be advised to utilize as much information from adult research as might be appropriate for use with children.

Patients' Rights

Most states have specific statutory law that spells out the rights of inpatients and residents in residential treatment programs. Clinicians working in these settings should be informed about the nature of these rights. Some of these rights are usually considered to be absolute (e.g., the right to practice religion), and others are considered to be conditional and can be taken away if proper procedures are followed (e.g., the right to communicate with others by telephone). If patients' rights are to be denied, then the procedures delineated in the state law must be followed. Most state laws cover the proper procedures to use when involuntary treatment is being sought, the guidelines for providing the least restrictive alternatives, and the rights of patients to refuse treatment. In some jurisdictions, patients must petition a court to refuse treatment; in other states, if a patient refuses, the mental health practitioner must petition the court to then provide treatment involuntarily. Clinicians must be informed in all these instances to avoid getting into difficulties. Whether clinicians are working in private practice or working in or consulting with community agencies, the laws on civil commitment are applicable uniformly.

Privacy, Confidentiality, and Privileged Communications

Most mental health professionals are well aware of the ethical issues involved in confidential communications with patients or clients, but the technical concepts of confidentiality and privileged communication are probably less well understood. *Confidentiality* generally refers to the ethical stricture that communications and information discussed with mental health professionals will not be disclosed or discussed further. In other words, confidentiality refers to a patient's right to privacy. This ethical principle is often codified in the ethical policies of the various professions. In some circumstances (e.g., where ethical principles or codes of professional conduct have been incorporated into state law), confidentiality may also have a legal basis for enforcement. That basis would be the statute governing practice of a profession and the administrative rules and regulations passed by the licensing board for that profession. It is important to know that rules and regulations bear the same force of law as the underlying statute for a particular profession.

Health Insurance Portability and Accountability Act

It is extremely important that clinicians be aware of the federal privacy standards that are a part of the Health Insurance Portability and Accountability Act (HIPAA) of 1996 (P.L. 104-191), which took effect on April 14, 2003. The clinician must know whether or not the HIPAA standards preempt state law with regard to privacy. As a general rule, the federal standard preempts state law wherever the state law is less stringent than the federal law. However, when the state law is more strict with regard to privacy issues than the federal law, state law will prevail. The behavior that triggers the HIPAA standards is the filing of an electronic claim for third-party reimbursement. If one's agency or clinic files insurance claims this way, then one is subject to these federal standards.

Privacy generally refers to the right of individuals to decide for themselves what they think, how they are going to behave, and what and how much they will share with others. People generally have an expectation of and a right to privacy unless their behavior or thinking has become so disordered as to interfere with others. Before clinicians can interfere with the privacy rights of individuals, clinicians must follow proper procedures that are usually codified in state laws dealing with items such as civil commitment of patients and reporting of abuse. Compulsory outpatient commitment is a related issue. In states where this provision applies, it is important to be aware of the requirements for such commitment, whether one's practice is in an agency, a community setting, or private practice.

In contrast to confidentiality, *privilege* is a relatively narrow concept. It specifically protects patients or clients from disclosure of information they have provided to mental health practitioners when the information is being requested for a legal proceeding of some kind. In general, privileged communication is covered in the licensing laws for mental health practitioners. Without a specific statutory basis, the communications between mental health practitioners and clients are generally not privileged. However, most state laws provide a variety of exceptions to privileged communication, and, in this area, certified or licensed clinicians must be aware of the limitations on privilege in their own state or jurisdiction.

Clinicians should also be aware that when they receive a subpoena regarding records and information they have, the subpoena does not eliminate the rules of confidentiality or privilege. Clinicians should generally assert privilege or the ethical stricture for confidentiality unless they have obtained a specific release of information from the client or patient. The court will then decide whether the information must be disclosed. A court-issued order to disclose protects the clinician who is disclosing the information. Mental health practitioners both in the private sector and in various agency settings need to be aware of other limitations of confidentiality and privileged communication that are found in most state laws and of laws that abrogate any privileges in their particular jurisdiction (e.g., almost all jurisdictions have child abuse reporting laws that take precedence over any statutes concerning confidentiality or privileged communication). Mental health practitioners are legally obligated to report when they have reason to believe that child abuse may be occurring.

It is also important to know whether the *duty to warn* is imposed by either statutory or case law in a particular jurisdiction (e.g., when a patient or client makes threats to a third person and the clinician believes that there is reason to take them seriously). Depending on the jurisdiction, such a situation may require the clinician or agency worker to report the threat to the intended victim or to a local police agency, to seek civil commitment of the patient, or to have some other type of action taken. Finally, there may be formal or legal repeal of the confidentiality or privileged communication statutes in some situations involving cases of domestic relations, such as when custody or visitation is an issue. In some jurisdictions, the mental health records of the parents or the child (or both) can be requested, and the party about whom the record has been made cannot assert either confidentiality or privilege to block its introduction into evidence.

Civil Commitment

Commitment laws vary widely from state to state, with the requirements for civil commitment being extremely liberal in some states and extremely conservative in others. Clinicians must understand the commitment law and its procedures for their particular jurisdiction. Failure to follow proper procedures can result in civil liability for false imprisonment or confinement. Most state laws have several different commitment procedures, ranging from emergency procedures to the more routine types of civil commitment. Mental health practitioners involved in these areas need to know the various deadlines and the types of evaluations that must be carried out within those deadlines. The rules regarding civil commitment of juveniles are significantly different from those involving adults. In 1967, the U.S. Supreme Court decided the case *In re Gault,* involving a 14-year-old juvenile who had made obscene telephone calls. The Supreme Court mandated due process for juveniles in the juvenile justice system because of the potential for abuse when courts used the "best interest" test (i.e., what was deemed in the juvenile's interest). However, in 1979, in *Parham v. J.R.*, the Supreme Court ruled that there was no requirement of an adversarial hearing for juvenile commitments, deciding that enough safeguards would exist if the request for civil commitment of a minor was presented to and examined by a "neutral fact finder." This case, against all expectations, upheld procedures that were being followed in the majority of states. *Parham* has been viewed as a victory for parental authority and for the emphasis on medical rather than judicial decision making. It was also seen as a retreat from procedural safeguards articulated in *Gault* for juvenile justice.

Most states have enacted laws consistent with the *Parham* case. Some state mental health systems and private hospitals have stricter rules than those articulated in *Parham*. Such procedures include obtaining the signature of juveniles over a certain age and in some instances meeting the standards for adult civil commitment for minors above a certain age. Therefore, clinicians must be aware of relevant state law and the rules of hospitals they might be working in or with because they must adhere to those laws and rules to avoid being held liable in a malpractice action.

Mental Health Professionals as Expert Witnesses in Court

Mental health professionals who are called to court to testify regarding various issues of concern to their patients should be aware of the changing landscape in U.S. law regarding the admissibility of mental health testimony. Until recently, the test for admissibility of scientific or professional evidence was the *Frye* test, wherein the court rejected evidence of the reliability of lie detector results because the scientific principles on which reliability was based were not well recognized in the community. The *Frye* test, also known as the general acceptance test, was a prerequisite to the admission of scientific evidence. In many subsequent cases, it was debated whether or not the *Frye* test had application to psychological evidence. In deciding the 1993 case of *Daubert v. Merrill Dow Pharmaceutical*, the U.S. Supreme Court held that rule 702 of the Federal Rules of Evidence (P.L. 93-595) superseded the *Frye* test. Thus the general acceptance standard for admissibility was changed. That court established a test based on four factors: 1) whether the scientific knowledge that would assist the trier of fact can be and has been tested, 2) whether the theory or technique had been subjected to peer review and publications, 3) the known or potential error rate of the technique, and 4) whether the science is identifiable and accepted within the scientific community. The court held that before admitting scientific testimony, a judge needed to consider these issues to weed out unreliable or "junk" science.

The next question that arose was whether courts would apply the *Daubert* standard to the social sciences. In *General Electric Co. v. Joiner* (1997), the Supreme Court decided that the studies on which experts had relied were not sufficient to support their conclusions and that exclusion of the testimony was warranted. In *Kumho Tire Co. v. Carmichael* (1999), the Supreme Court extended *Daubert* to opinion testimony of other experts who are not scientists. It was generally accepted that clinicians and researchers would now find themselves held to a higher standard before being allowed to present expert testimony regarding their assessments and treatments. Since then, a number of state courts have explicitly opted to follow the *Daubert* rule, and at least 27 states have decided that the standards are either helpful or controlling. Eleven states actually rejected *Daubert* and continue to use *Frye*. Therefore, it is extremely important that mental health professionals know the rules for their jurisdiction. Federal evidence rule 702 was modified to reflect the Supreme Court's holdings in the three cases described above:

> If the scientific, technical, or other specialized knowledge will assist the trier of fact to understand the evidence or to determine a fact in issue, a witness qualified as an expert by knowledge, skill, experience, training, or education may testify thereto in the form of an opinion or otherwise, if (1) the testimony is based upon sufficient facts or data, (2) the testimony is the product of reliable principles and methods, and (3) the witness has applied the principles and methods reliably to the facts of the case. (P.L. 93-595, amended April 17, 2000; effective December 1, 2000)

This new version of the rule does not exactly reference the four *Daubert* standards, but it does require that the underlying facts or data an expert is relying on are sufficient to support the opinion and that the principles and methods on which the data are based be applied reliably to the facts of the particular case. Mental health professionals need to be aware that if a particular state enacts the uniform rule, they will then be held to that standard. Meanwhile, mental health professionals who testify in court should be aware that they should have some understanding of the underlying bases—particularly research, if it exists—for any opinion that they give. It is irresponsible for experts to rely only on their own clinical experience if there is a database or research literature dealing with the issue in question. In fact, the opinion testimony may be excluded unless the expert knows the underlying research.

■ CONCLUSIONS

The community mental health professional may find the following list of key law-related concepts handy for ready reference:

- *Scope of practice:* Keep abreast of state law defining one's scope of practice, paying particular attention to the issues of whether diagnosis and treatment of mental disorders is permitted and whether any requirements for supervision exist.
- *Malpractice:* Be aware of the major areas of potential malpractice, be sure to do what evidence-based practice suggests in each case, and avoid doing anything that could lead to a complaint being filed.
- *Competency:* Because evidence-based practice is increasingly becoming the norm in mental health care, make diligent efforts to keep abreast of changing standards of care for the various diagnostic categories of patients.
- *Patients' rights:* Always know the specific rights that patients retain when hospitalized or in residential programs. Be particularly sensitive to the state laws defining the least-restrictive treatment requirement and of patients' rights to refuse treatments under certain conditions of state law.
- *Privacy, confidentiality, and privileged communications:* Know the distinctions between these concepts and follow existing ethical or legal requirements. Be aware of the additional and more stringent requirements engendered by HIPAA. Attend mandatory compliance training programs dealing with HIPAA on a yearly basis and be especially sensitive to the heightened privacy requirements now in existence.
- *Civil commitment:* Be aware of state law controlling commitment of juveniles, as well as specific policies of the employer that may grant juveniles more rights than the law requires.
- *Expert witness testimony:* Know the current legal standards for admissibility of expert testimony and any scientific or research evidence available to support the opinions of expert clinicians testifying in court.

This chapter covers some of the possible areas for legal involvement of mental health practitioners working in community settings. For general information on particular jurisdictions, readers are referred to the Law and Mental Health Professionals series published by the American Psychological Association. This series will eventually include a volume for each state, covering various areas of mental health law; each volume will be periodically updated. Several state volumes have been completed, and those for other states are near completion. Practitioners today must be aware of the laws that affect the various areas in which they practice. Practicing without an awareness of the legal issues impinging on one's practice could subject the clinician to serious legal penalties if mistakes are made, even inadvertently. It is also important that mental health practitioners consult with an attorney—either the attorney for the agency where one is employed or one's private attorney—whenever questions arise about the legal aspects of some clinical practice. Legal issues and principles apply uniformly to clinicians whether they work within an agency or are consulting to an agency. The consultation literature distinguishes between consultants and supervisors, with the emphasis on consultants not being in a supervisory role. However, consultants likely would be held to whatever legal standards or standards of care that exist, regardless of this fine distinction in the clinical literature. It is also important to emphasize that there is no difference among community practice, hospital practice, and private practice regarding the need for clinicians in each of these areas to be aware of the law and its applicability to them in their particular circumstance. The same general principles apply to the clinician testifying in court, whether he or she is an employee of an agency or a consultant to a community agency. The general legal principles regarding competence to testify as well as issues of credibility of witnesses will apply regardless of the clinician's status.

■ REFERENCES

Ceci SJ, Bruck M: Jeopardy in the Courtroom: A Scientific Analysis of Children's Testimony. Washington, DC, American Psychological Association, 1995

Daubert v Merrill Dow Pharmaceutical, 509 US 579, 1993

Federal Rules of Evidence, Pub. L. No. 93-595

General Electric Co. v Joiner, 522 US 136, 1997

Health Insurance Portability and Accountability Act of 1996, Pub. L. No. 104-191

In re Gault, 387 US 1, 1967

Kumho Tire Co. v Carmichael, 526 US 137, 1999

Landeros v Flood, 551 P2d 389, 1976

Lawlor RJ: The expert witness in child sexual abuse cases: a clinician's view, in Expert Witnesses in Child Abuse Cases: What Can and Should Be Said in Court. Edited by Ceci SJ, Hembrooke H. Washington, DC, American Psychological Association, 1998, pp 105–122

Mossman D: Assessing predictions of violence: being accurate about accuracy. J Consult Clin Psychol 62:783–792, 1994

Otto R: The prediction of dangerous behavior: a review and analysis of "second generation" research. Forensic Reports 5:103–133, 1992

Parham v J.R., 442 US 584, 1979

Wickline v California, 228 Cal Rptr 661 (Cal Ct App 1986)

Wilson v Blue Cross of Southern California, 271 Cal Rptr 876 (Cal Ct App 1990)

4 PRACTICAL ASPECTS OF RURAL MENTAL HEALTH CARE

Stuart Copans, M.D.

This chapter is intended to help mental health practitioners who are living or working in a rural area with some of the problems they may encounter and to help those considering a move to a rural area to make a more informed decision about such a move. In the practice of rural mental health care, some general principles need to be taken into account in addition to crucial specifics that vary from one rural area to another. The geography, demography, ethnic and cultural heritage, financial arrangements, and transportation systems vary widely in different rural areas. Rural areas have some features in common, however. Any mental health practitioner moving to such an area must be prepared to consider the following:

- In most rural areas, there are significant shortages of mental health professionals. You will be called on to do more than you think you are capable of, both in numbers of cases and in the range of problems that arise.
- As a practitioner in a rural area, you will be a public figure, as will your family.
- Relationships in rural areas are crucial. This includes both personal relationships and relationships with other health care and mental health care providers. If you are more interested in applying techniques and performing procedures than in dealing with people, then you may want to stay in an urban environment.

- Most rural areas include a variety of racial, religious, and ethnic groups. Good mental health care involves developing a sensitivity and knowledge base about these groups and about their histories, heritage, belief systems, and role in the community. If you have strong negative feelings about any religious, racial, or ethnic groups, you may wish to remain in an urban area where you can limit your practice.
- Boundary issues and confidentiality are extraordinarily important and at times difficult. They can be managed by using a combination of ethics, law, and common sense and by sharing your dilemmas with patients and their families so that you can find mutually acceptable arrangements.
- Standards of practice must be adapted to rural realities. However, it is important not to compromise quality of care too easily. When compromises are necessary, inform the family so they can share in the decisions.
- The needs for clinical services and for generating income may create pressures to spend almost all of your time in direct patient care. Don't succumb! You need to function as part of a team, and in particular as part of a team with a shared vision of good clinical care. That will not happen unless the team has time to meet and talk about shared cases and problematic cases. You may want to reconsider or decline working in an agency that does not expect members of its child mental health team to meet on an ongoing and regular basis.
- Many child mental health care providers move away from rural areas because they found they were unable to make an adequate living. You do yourself, your patients, and the agencies you contract with a disservice if you agree to a level of reimbursement that results in your moving away after 6 months.

Although there may seem to be few geographic similarities between the wide-open, sparsely populated areas of West Texas; the little Appalachian valleys of West Virginia; and the large quilt-work farms of the Midwestern prairies, they are all united by the concept that (as the saying goes) "you can't get there from here." Geography often creates real obstacles that affect the structure of communities, and it also affect your ability to get to patients and their ability to get to you. Ethnic and cultural diversities represent another rural characteristic. Each rural area may have its own set of cultures, and those cultures are often patchworks that must be studied to be understood. To practice rural mental health care, you need to know your community and to understand the cultural values and the geography that help create it (Hill and Fraser 1995). A good way to learn about both the geography and the cultures is to visit the homes of your patients as part of your initial assessment. Although such visits are difficult to justify in the current cost-conscious climate, you should make a serious effort to do some visits, at least in your initial few months in a new community.

An outline of a home visit (Copans 1997a) can be summarized as follows:

1. Explain to the family that to get to know them and their neighborhood better, you would like to visit them at their home and have a meal with them.
2. Work out a mutually convenient date and get detailed directions.
3. When you go on the visit, allow time to get a sense of the neighborhood.
4. When you arrive, ask for a tour. If there is a garden, a barn, or animals, ask if you can see them. Note what the family is particularly proud of. Ask the child to show you where he or she sleeps and to show you any special things or special places the child would like you to see.
5. When leaving, thank the family for the dinner and compliment them on their special things and on areas of family strength you have noticed.
6. That evening, if possible, or at latest the next day, write down your observations and impressions in detail.

In working with rural families, time is often your greatest asset. Although urban families often want their problems fixed immediately, rural families may be used to and accepting of a different pace; the opportunity to observe and monitor over time allows you to clarify a diagnosis without your observations being confounded by the effects of psychotropic medication. Time can be particularly helpful when children present with symptoms of attention-deficit/hyperactivity disorder (ADHD), because the differential diagnosis is broad and includes some diagnoses—such as posttraumatic stress disorder, anxiety disorders, or affective disorders—that may be difficult to detect because of family secrecy or shame.

■ RURAL PRACTICE

Rural Values

Besides the multiple cultures that make up a rural area, some authors have described a set of values that they argue are shared by residents in many rural areas (Bachrach 1983; Cook et al. 1998; Flaskerud and Kviz 1983). These authors believe that although rural residents differ greatly in their ethnic backgrounds, socioeconomic makeup, and belief systems, they share commonalities, which include the following:

* *Individualism:* A strong belief in the right to act as an individual and a rejection of help from the community or any governmental agency. This trait can be harnessed to help with treatment.
* *Family cohesiveness:* A strong tendency to seek help within the family and to protect the family from what are perceived as outside meddlers. It is therefore crucial to present family therapy in a way that utilizes this tendency and does not conflict with it.

- *Independence:* Rural individuals have a need to feel that they control their life and their behavior. Rural mental health practitioners should talk about the way in which untreated illness may make people more dependent than if they obtain the necessary treatment.

- *Distrust of outsiders:* Outsiders often must prove themselves before being accepted.

- *A powerful work orientation:* This orientation may make it hard for many rural families to participate in therapy during the usual hours. When family members say they cannot miss work for family therapy, it is not necessarily resistance. Some flexibility about scheduling is crucial for therapists performing rural work.

- *Avoiding conflict:* The strongly held notion that it is best to avoid conflict may make the process of therapy difficult. This notion is encapsulated in rural proverbs (e.g., the Vermont aphorism, "Never get in a pissing contest with a skunk"; or the South Carolina variant, "Never wrestle with a pig—you both get dirty, and the pig likes it"). However, these proverbs can be used to point out that sometimes "pigs" and "skunks" need limits, and that shooting them (one rural approach to avoiding conflict) is not the recommended remedy if the animals in the proverbs refer to the family's teenage children.

Collaborations and Clinical Practice

In rural areas, consultation and collaboration are particularly important and all too often are underutilized. Collaborative teams are particularly important in the treatment of many problems in children and adolescents, such as pervasive developmental disorders or attention-deficit disorders (especially when they are comorbid with learning deficits or other disruptive disorders).

ADHD and Pervasive Developmental Disorder: Multidisciplinary Approaches for Effective and Cost-Efficient Collaboration

Important areas for collaboration include the diagnosis and treatment of ADHD and pervasive developmental disorder. Inattention or hyperactivity in school has many causes: depression; learning difficulties; malnutrition or infections; preoccupation because of difficulties at home; brain disorders such as brain tumors and Arnold-Chiari malformation; or even psychotic, manic, or pervasive developmental disorders. It is important that a diagnosis of ADHD be made only after a careful assessment of physical and psychological symptoms (Bennett et al. 1998). In many rural areas, the diagnosis of ADHD is based on a telephone call from the teacher to the parents, and treatment consists of a prescription for stimulant medication. Although it does lead to improvement, this community treatment model is not as effective as medication management by a child psychiatrist (consisting of monthly half-hour meetings with parent and child and regular use of ADHD scales to monitor progress), behavioral interventions with parents and teachers, or a combination of medication and behavioral treatments. Evaluation, as performed in most psychiatric settings, should include a physical examination, cognitive testing (because unrecognized learning disabilities may often appear to be inattention), and an assessment of the family and the classroom. Although resources are limited in rural areas, it is usually possible for a school system to put together a local team to carry out evaluations and to work with parents, teachers, and pediatricians to develop comprehensive treatment plans. Such a team can either include a child psychiatrist or establish contact with one to help in the development of evaluation and treatment protocols. The child psychiatrist can work with the team to evaluate children who do not respond to the initial intervention or who seem to have problems that go beyond a simple case of ADHD. Recent large-scale studies seem to clearly indicate that children who have ADHD in addition to other psychiatric diagnoses benefit more from an approach that combines careful monitoring of medication by a child psychiatrist with work with both family members and teachers.

This approach, in which a multidisciplinary team together works out a protocol that helps clarify when each professional needs to be involved, can be particularly helpful in the treatment of children with pervasive developmental disorder. The team might meet as a whole infrequently, although it should meet at least quarterly to review cases or hear an educational presentation. Individual children living in widely separated communities could be followed up by subsets of the team. This group can be called in, referred to, or consulted by telephone as needed. Team members would have other primary jobs and would set aside a certain number of hours to work with the team. This model can help involve relatively distant professionals, who can be available by telephone for support or to help in making decisions about referral when questions come up. Members of the interdisciplinary team can improve their work together and can help work with a distant consultant by the use of agreed-on ways of collecting and displaying data, such as Conners' Rating Scales (Conners 1997) or the Beck Depression Inventory (Beck 1993).

With its chronological display of the patient's life beginning at or before conception and continuing through the present, the Meyerian Life Chart can serve as a unifying device (Copans 1997a). The graphic display of all this information can help to clarify discrepancies between the histories obtained by different members of the treatment team and can create a common body of knowledge that leads to clearer communication between team members and between the team and the patient or family (Cook et al. 1998).

Particularly Difficult Issues

Numerous difficult issues that require attention include the following:

- Dealing with limited resources
- Utilizing available resources
- Boundaries, confidentiality, and conflicts of interest
- Continuing education, professional organizations, and support
- Your role in the community
- Taking care of yourself and your family
- Facing the issue of finances and case loads
- Other practicalities
- Relocation

Dealing With Limited Resources

At times, certain tests or therapies might not be available in rural areas, or if they are available, transportation or cost may be insurmountable barriers. Making the choice between the need for a service and its relative expense is often difficult. Examples are 1) whether to use what you consider an optimal medication if it is excessively expensive or extremely complicated (because of the need to measure blood levels or to check blood counts), 2) whether to use family therapy when the nearest family therapist is an hour's drive away, or 3) whether to see a child monthly instead of weekly when transportation issues make weekly visits unreasonable. Decisions about restricting treatments due to scarcity of resources or about the extent to which standards of care could be compromised because of financial considerations must be shared with families. Such circumstances must be brought to the attention of both administrators and legislators. As mental health care moves from a bimodal model, primarily consisting of outpatient and hospital services, to an array of services including inpatient services, intensive day treatment/partial hospitalization, residential care, outpatient services, and case management, the rural system will experience considerable stress. The impact on rural mental health care—where the low volume of patients and transportation problems make the development of intensive day services or even outpatient group therapy difficult or impossible—can be particularly limiting. **We cannot allow managed care organizations to avoid paying for care when they approve only levels of care and services that are not available.**

Utilizing Available Resources

The rural child and adolescent mental health professional has the opportunity to apply creative solutions to the multiple problems and barriers described. This means considering what is available, what is affordable, and what is accessible.

Boundaries, Confidentiality, and Conflicts of Interest

Boundaries and confidentiality are significant problems in a rural practice. New rules need to be developed when your son's classmate tells your son that he is your patient or when your children are on a Little League team with your patient. Although clearly, we cannot violate a patient's rights by breaking confidentiality, in many ways our encounters with patients in these other settings give us a chance to reinforce our message that mental illness is not stigmatizing. A surgeon does not discuss a patient's appendectomy when he sees her at a cocktail party, but neither does he feel that ordinary social interactions must be avoided because of their doctor–patient relationship. It is important to discuss with patients how they would like you to act when you encounter them in a social setting—and then to act accordingly (Schetky 1995). An additional problem faced by rural mental health workers is the knowledge that they have about the people they see. It is sometimes helpful to be direct with the parents about what you have already heard about them. At other times, it is important to have boundaries not only between you and your patients but also within your mind, so that you can wall off whatever you know and approach the evaluation with an open mind (Copans and Racusin 1983). How you decide the course to take in a given evaluation is beyond the scope of this chapter. It is learned through years of rural practice, by learning from occasional mistakes, and by having discussions with colleagues.

Continuing Education, Professional Organizations, and Support

When you practice in a rural area, it is crucial that you continue your education, continue your involvement with professional organizations, and develop a support network of your peers. Attending professional education meetings is particularly important precisely because doing so is difficult and because you are so isolated. As a rural practitioner, you should have two professional support groups: a multidisciplinary local support group of other mental health practitioners and a support group of others from your discipline whom you can call and consult with. If possible, you should teach and should arrange to have social work students, medical students, residents, psychology interns, and child psychiatry nursing students work with you. Teach a course on child development, psychopathology, the consultation process, or a related topic area at the local community college. Write articles, present at meetings, or join a professional network to study outcomes of practice. These strategies can create a whole new appreciation for your work and at the same time can assist you in improving your practice and your knowledge base.

Your Role in the Community

As a rural child mental health professional, you are living in a fishbowl. To maintain your credibility, you will need to adapt to the norms of the community (Petti 1997). You have the potential to contribute to the community in many ways; at the same time, it is wise to tread slowly. People in the rural community care less about the fact that you graduated with high honors than that you were able to help their neighbor's child. Learn to listen in town meetings before you speak, and for the first few years don't say much. If living modestly and morally (as defined by the community) is a burden, you may not want to live in a rural area, or you may want to find one that has values compatible with your own. Take an active part in community life. Shop locally whenever you can, and think of the extra few dollars it is likely to cost as a donation to the viability of the town, or perhaps as a way of priming the pump from which you too draw your water.

Taking Care of Yourself and Your Family

Being married to a saint, or having one for a father or mother, can be rough. To avoid putting your family through such hardship, make sure that you sometimes put your children and your marriage ahead of your patients in your priority system. Reschedule patients so you can see your daughter play in the regional championships. Make sure you take time off and go somewhere where you can't be reached. Federal regulations require bankers to take a 2-week vacation every year and stay away from the bank for the whole period. Similar rules should exist for rural therapists. People can survive without you, and if you can't survive without taking care of them, you are not taking good care of them. You owe it to your patients as well as to your family and yourself to take regular vacations.

Finances and Case Loads

Finances are often a problem for rural mental health professionals and are usually an even bigger problem for those working in child and adolescent mental health. The incidence of poverty is higher in rural areas. As a result, more patients are eligible for Medicaid, which often reimburses at low rates. As a child mental health professional with specialized skills—for example, a speech and language therapist, a psychologist, a clinical nurse specialist, or a child psychiatrist—you may find that any given agency cannot justify hiring you full-time. You may need to contract with a variety of agencies to put together a full-time job. Rural agencies often assume that part-time workers should cost less than full-time workers. However, it is critical that rural mental health professionals and administrators keep the big picture in mind, particularly when contracting for services.

For several reasons, agencies may have to pay as much as 40% of a yearly salary for a 1-day-a-week employee. Such employees may be spending 20%–30% of their time driving between widely separated work sites and in addition are responsible for their own health insurance, dental insurance, malpractice insurance, sick days, disability, Social Security, life insurance, retirement, continuing education, vacations, association memberships, communication system, and transportation. The different agencies should share responsibility in compensating for the employee's transportation time. Although administrators' initial reaction to sharing this cost may be one of shock, it is important for them to realize the advantages this sharing provides them. The contract involves no benefits (which typically add 25%–40% to the cost of a full-time employee), no risk (such as sick days or disability), and no costs for space or secretarial support on the days the part-time professionals are not working there. Part-time workers generally devote a much higher percentage of their time to direct service than full-time employees. Thus these amounts may seem much less unreasonable.

The dilemma of services that are not reimbursed is a practical dilemma for all professionals working with youngsters—but is especially difficult for rural child mental health professionals and their administrators, because insurance will not pay for collateral contacts, school visits, or travel time. One solution devised by rural practitioners is to schedule a 1-hour visit with a child. Some of that time is spent in individual work with the child, some with the parents, and some in contacting other individuals involved in the child's case while the child continues playing or drawing in the office.

Another financial dilemma in rural areas is the problem of missed appointments. Because of time, distance, weather, and transportation problems, missed appointments are more common in rural areas. Typically, missed appointments are not reimbursed. Although terminating treatment might seem justified with an adult who frequently does not show up for appointments, terminating treatment is harder with children, because the children with unreliable parents are often the ones most in need of treatment. If good care is to be provided, rural child mental health workers need to have significantly lower case loads than are typically assigned to those working with adults. Although the difference in time demands between child and adult cases also applies in urban and suburban clinics, the nature of rural communities and rural geography makes collateral contacts in rural areas even more important and more difficult.

Other Practicalities

In rural areas, it is important to learn to talk in language that will be understood. Use local proverbs or stories to make your interpretations.

New technologies such as telemedicine and computerized follow-up calls may make positive contributions to the practice of rural mental health. These technologies could also have negative effects if they lead to increased separation of the mental health professionals from the patients and communities they are serving. As we incorporate these new technologies into our rural practices, we must continue to practice in ways that maintain our contact with and knowledge of the families and communities that our patients are part of, because personal involvement continues to be important in rural areas. Using these technologies to facilitate meetings of interdisciplinary teams or to facilitate continuing education, supervision, consultation, or follow-up with distant patients when transportation is a problem may help overcome some of the problems of distance, as long as we maintain our human connections.

Time spent driving is a joy and hardship of rural practice. Falling asleep is a big danger when working hard and driving far, so you need to develop some techniques for staying awake. Which muscles can you tense and then relax while driving? Learn to pull over and take 10-minute catnaps. Always carry a full thermos of hot coffee. Sometimes open the windows, let in the cold air, and recite poetry. There are also ways to use driving time. Because using a cellular phone significantly increases the accident rate, I recommend not using one while driving. Some newer car phones with microphones and speakers built into the car may not have the same effect on accident rates as those that are hand held. If so, use of such a phone would make it possible to use driving time to return calls and to follow up on patients seen during the day. I listen to continuing-education tapes and sometimes listen to tapes of novels or nonfiction books. One agency sent me a cassette containing a case description of the patient I was about to see; I was able to play the cassette in the car on my way to the agency.

How to say no—and when not to—probably constitute the most important judgments—and the most difficult ones—you will have to make as a rural mental health practitioner. Balancing your ethical responsibilities, political considerations, financial considerations, and need to save time for yourself and your family is a skill you will learn only by trial and error. Those who never say little noes often end up saying a big *no* by moving away. Your telephone is a blessing and a curse. It can help you follow up with patients, stay in contact with referral sources, and phone in prescriptions, but it can give people unprotected access to you. It can let your office work follow you home so that your work invades your family life, and it can both pressure you and tempt you to do things over the phone that should be done face to face. Telephone contact is almost never reimbursable, so it can take up an immense amount of your time without generating any income. In rural communities, answering services may be hard to use because of problems of confidentiality. The telephone is another area where learning to say no is a crucial part of survival in rural practice. With voice mail and caller identification, you should be able to eat dinner with your family without interruption. If you find yourself unable to stop taking calls, seek out some supervision or even some therapy.

Relocation

For those of you from urban areas, I encourage you to explore the possibilities of a rural practice. If you are married or have children, explore the possibilities together with your family. Dragging them, kicking and screaming, to a better life in a pastoral setting is not likely to work (Copans 1997b; McCollum et al. 1996). On the other hand, for many families who make the decision to leave "civilization" behind and join those of us who are willing to trade some of our privacy and anonymity for community, intimacy, and a different pace of life—living and working in rural areas, choosing "the path less traveled by"—has indeed "made all the difference." In a rural setting, your skills will be needed, useful, and appreciated.

▍ CONCLUSIONS

For many of us who grew up and live and work in rural areas, the satisfaction of being a valued member of a small community and of being able to help children in areas where our services are scarce and are needed far outweighs the disadvantages.

▍ REFERENCES

Bachrach LL: Psychiatric services in rural areas: a sociological overview. Hosp Community Psychiatry 34:215–225, 1983

Beck AT: Beck Depression Inventory (BDI) Manual, 2nd Edition. San Antonio, TX, Psychological Corporation, 1993

Bennett R, Knorr W, Copans SA: Which of these children has AD/HD? the answer may surprise you. Reaching Today's Youth 2:6–10, 1998

Conners CK: Conners' Rating Scales–Revised, Technical Manual. North Tonawanda, NY, 1997

Cook AD, Copans SA, Schetky DH: Psychiatric treatment of children and adolescents in rural communities: myths and realities. Child Adolesc Psychiatr Clin N Am 7:673–690, 1998

Copans SA: Immigrant and refugee children, in Handbook of Child and Adolescent Psychiatry, Vol 4: Varieties of Development. Edited by Alessi NE (Noshpitz JD, ed in chief). New York, Wiley, 1997a, pp 619–631

Copans SA: When children relocate, in Handbook of Child and Adolescent Psychiatry, Vol 4: Varieties of Development. Edited by Alessi NE (Noshpitz JD, ed in chief). New York, Wiley, 1997b, pp 631–638

Copans SA, Racusin R: Rural child psychiatry. J Am Acad Child Psychiatry 22:184–190, 1983

Flaskerud JH, Kviz FJ: Rural attitudes toward and knowledge of mental illness and treatment resources. Hosp Community Psychiatry 34:229–233, 1983

Hill CE, Fraser GJ: Local knowledge and rural mental health reform. Community Ment Health J 31:553–568, 1995

McCollum A, Jensen N, Copans SA: Smart Moves: Your Guide Through the Emotional Maze of Relocation. Lyme, NH, Smith and Kraus, 1996

Petti TA: The rural child, in Handbook of Child and Adolescent Psychiatry, Vol 4: Varieties of Development. Edited by Alessi NE (Noshpitz JD, ed in chief). New York, Wiley, 1997, pp 220–228

Schetky D: Boundaries in child and adolescent psychiatry. Child Adolesc Psychiatr Clin N Am 4:769–778, 1995

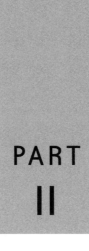

PART
II

The Core Mental Health
Professionals

5 | ROLE OF THE CHILD AND ADOLESCENT PSYCHIATRIST

John M. Diamond, M.D.

Judith Doğin, M.D.

Physicians are trained to treat medical problems in a unique doctor–patient relationship. Child and adolescent psychiatrists are trained within this medical model to evaluate, diagnose, and treat mental disorders in their patients. Child and adolescent psychiatrists are often motivated to participate actively in community practice and consultation because mental health services delivered in traditional outpatient settings do not reach the vast majority of those who have psychiatric disorders. Because of the high prevalence of psychiatric disorders and the shortage of child and adolescent psychiatrists, it is imperative that the psychiatrists' role be understood by all professionals working in the public sector (or planning to do so) and that the psychiatrists' training reflect the need for their services. This chapter emphasizes the manner in which child and adolescent psychiatrists are trained for community-based practice, administration, and consultation and delineates their roles in community settings.

Child and adolescent psychiatrists in training have already obtained a bachelor's degree and medical school training that emphasizes the medical model (i.e., working to develop a diagnosis that serves as a hypothesis and then testing that hypothesis by monitoring the clinical course or intervening with treatment that is expected to improve the course of illness). They have become well versed in identifying early normal and pathological development of the body and the mind, in administering physical and mental status examinations, and in working within a complex system of service delivery (i.e., hospitals and clinic settings). In their training in general psychiatry and child and adolescent psychiatry, they develop the skills to integrate biological, psychological, and social perspectives, methods, and tools for the evaluation and treatment of children and adolescents and their families. When trainees have mastered the challenges of comprehensive evaluation, psychopharmacological and psychological treatment, and social support of youths and families, they are introduced to the techniques of consultation to agencies and systems. The principles of collaboration with other professionals in the care of youths in pediatric, school, forensic, and community health and mental health centers and other community settings are taught through didactic seminars and supervised clinical experiences.

The supervised experiences are of varying duration and intensity and are usually conducted in schools but also take place in community mental health centers (CMHCs), juvenile courts or detention centers, child welfare agencies, day care programs, and residential treatment centers or group homes. In this process, child and adolescent psychiatrists learn to appreciate the unique needs of nontraditional mental health programs and of families who come from varied cultural, religious, and socioeconomic backgrounds. Community psychiatry training prepares child and adolescent psychiatrists to care for youths and families touched by psychiatric disturbance and the impact of poverty or other social and demographic factors in rural and urban community settings. Trainees learn to understand the impact of poverty on development, family functioning, and behavioral health within the community system of health and human services. They are exposed to concepts such as coordinated systems of care and are taught about the Child and Adolescent Service System Program and related funding programs that have allowed states to begin planning and developing systems of care (see Stroul and Friedman 1986). Through didactic exercises, trainees consider issues related to systems development and functioning and the theory and practice of mental health consultation (see Chapter 1, "Working Within Communities").

▌ THE CHILD AND ADOLESCENT PSYCHIATRIST IN COMMUNITY SETTINGS

Community settings offer myriad opportunities for child and adolescent psychiatrists to put into practice the skills they have honed through years of education and training. This background includes earning a bachelor's degree and a medical degree and completing a postgraduate medical residency in psychiatry and then a specialized postgraduate medical residency in child and adolescent psychiatry. A partial list of activities of child and adolescent psychiatrists follows:

- Integrate biological, psychological, and social perspectives
- Clinically evaluate children and adolescents and their families
- Establish diagnoses
- Develop treatment plans
- Treat psychiatric disorders
- Provide consultation to health care professionals and professionals in pediatric, school, forensic, and other community settings

Role of Child and Adolescent Psychiatrists Across Community Settings

The community practice of child and adolescent psychiatry is often considered to be practice in a CMHC (also called a catchment area or area program). The role is undergoing an evolution, and psychiatrists are practicing in and consulting to multiple agencies within the human service system universe. Although these agencies differ from state to state, they are generally part of local government, such as counties or groups of counties. Child and adolescent psychiatrists may be employed full-time by an agency or may provide service on a part-time basis. Roles vary across these settings, as noted in the other chapters in this book. The spectrum of clinical practice ranges from administration to direct care of the patient, client, or student; and from program direction to the various types of consultation.

The current practice of mental health care in community settings differs from that originally practiced in child guidance centers of the past. Although the treatment team is still the model for clinical practice, practice is no longer office bound. As psychopharmacology has risen to the forefront of clinical practice, therapy or counseling in community public settings is generally performed by other mental health professionals—increasingly so as clinical and agency programs are being fiscally strained. Psychiatrists generally provide services for which external funding is available—services that in most settings are currently limited to diagnostic assessments and medication management. This situation has created dilemmas for child and adolescent psychiatrists who wish to practice in a scientific and ethical manner and to alleviate the pain and suffering of their patients and their patients' family members. The particular expertise of child and adolescent psychiatrists lies in the application of the biopsychosocial model. Prescribing and monitoring the use of psychotropic medication is one mainstay of that approach. But the literature is equivocal on the effectiveness of psychopharmacological treatment for many disorders of children and adolescents and on the effectiveness of split treatment between psychiatrists and other mental health professionals. At the time of this writing, the documented effectiveness of psychotropic medication is limited, whereas the public is more demanding of drug treatment. As child and adolescent psychiatrists choose to apply evidence-based treatment to psychopharmacological practice, they find few randomized, double-blind trials on which to build rational treatment plans. So they employ the best available evidence and practice parameters as guides. The clinician must be aware of the limited evidence base and must obtain clear informed consent. The child and family should be part of the decision making and should be provided with knowledge about relevant risks and benefits. Because few medications have received approval from the U.S. Food and Drug Administration for childhood indications, the informing and decision-making process must also be understood by administrators as a significant reason that appointments for children and families require additional time.

Many child and adolescent psychiatrists recognize that they must play a greater role in the day-to-day operation of certain programs and in program development. This role may include clinical staffing or case review. In some centers the psychiatrists evaluate every new intake. Other centers limit the involvement of psychiatrists to clinical review and direct evaluation of a portion of the cases reviewed. Managed care is increasing its demand for clinical accountability, and psychiatrists may need to be present when services are delivered to sign off on billing forms. Psychiatrists must understand that their signature implies direct patient contact, which often constitutes a requirement to bill. Psychiatrists may also be asked to review treatment plans. For billing purposes, this task may be approached as a form of consultee-centered consultation, as supervision, or as a clinical or administrative role. Psychiatrists need to be certain that the role is clear before providing a signature, because unless it is otherwise specified, the signature of a psychiatrist on a clinical document implies that the psychiatrist has prepared the document personally, has had personal contact with the patient, and takes responsibility for the content of the document (American Academy of Child and Adolescent Psychiatry 1996). In signing a treatment plan without seeing the client, the psychiatrist assumes responsibility for the defined treatment plan, which should be clearly configured and carried out by other members of the treatment team. Providing a signature denotes that one has discussed the case and endorses the treatment plan. If the signature reflects that the psychiatrist is providing supervision, then the supervisee's name and role should also appear on the document. The psychiatrist who is unfamiliar with an agency, a team, or its resources assumes enormous risk in signing treatment plans. The well-versed psychiatrist makes informed and ethical decisions when signing a document. This process comprises legal, fiscal, clinical, liability, and ethical concerns.

Collaboration with nonmedical clinicians has become a rather universal method of practice in CMHCs. The clinician, often the patient's psychotherapist or case manager, may be present during a medication evaluation. This arrangement facilitates communication about a patient but can lead to new administrative concerns when it is not permissible for two clinicians to be reimbursed for the same time. Accurate charting improves communication; however, most clinicians find it an unsatisfactory method of promoting clinical communication. A cost-effective model that clinicians find satisfying has yet to be disseminated and accepted.

Psychiatrists are generally most satisfied working in agencies where adequate support staff ensure prompt charting and filing and are available for collaboration. The arrangement may be most satisfying when therapists or case managers are not dependent on client billing for services; school counselors, social workers and social psychologists, social workers in social service departments, and even probation officers are usually salaried and are not dependent on clinical income production. In these settings, their presence during psychiatric appointments allows for modeling as well as enhanced collaboration.

Roles of Child and Adolescent Psychiatrists Within Agencies

The role of the child and adolescent psychiatrist varies from agency to agency depending on the individual psychiatrist and the structure of the agency. The role of the child and adolescent psychiatrist generally involves a blending of direct patient care, consultation, and administrative tasks:

Direct care of patients

- Clinical evaluation
- Medication management or pharmacotherapy
- Psychotherapy (individual, group, family)

Consultation

- Client centered
- Administrative

Administration of clinical programs

- Clinical practice development and oversight
- Leadership of interdisciplinary treatment teams
- Liaison with managed care organizations and payers
- Oversight of quality improvement activities

With community systems of care crossing agency boundaries, child and adolescent psychiatrists are also defining new roles in these systems. These psychiatrists often find themselves working within school systems, social service agencies, and juvenile justice departments and cast into unconventional roles in the different agencies. Functioning more as consultants or system advocates, they facilitate interagency coordination of care for youths and their families. Systems of care are usually driven by case management; their focus is on providing wraparound services to improve functional abilities. Child and adolescent psychiatrists need to interact with case managers, who are seldom versed in the medical model. Because case managers often seek nontraditional services for children, child and adolescent psychiatrists need to understand how these alternative services can promote improved mental health. The child and adolescent psychiatrist may also have a role in quality assurance. Consultation and supervision can be used to ensure appropriate services and monitor clinical efficacy. The following vignette illustrates the role of the child and adolescent psychiatrist in a system of care:

> A 9-year-old boy was in the custody of his mother, an active substance abuser, but lived with his maternal grandmother. The state department of social services had been investigating the family. The boy was referred to the CMHC by his teacher for evaluation of very active and impulsive behavior, but he missed two appointments for medication evaluation. After the third missed appointment, the psychiatrist, the resident, and the case manager made a trip to the grandmother's house with the intention of evaluating the child in his home, but the boy was not there. The clinic workers were able to meet with the boy's grandmother to discuss the family's needs and develop a strength-based treatment plan. Volunteers from the family's church provided transportation, and a member of the extended family helped the child further develop his artistic interests. This led to a meeting of all interested parties; the family and the child eventually viewed the department of social services as an ally because the caseworker had helped promote the treatment plan. The extended family member became an advocate for the child and provided a liaison to the school, which was able to increase artistic expression as part of the boy's individual education plan.

The concern in managed care organizations regarding treatment effectiveness has increased the need for accountability. The results of treatment effectiveness studies may eventually direct treatment planning, but a current need exists for monitoring symptom change and improved functioning. This need has become a quality assurance concern. In reviewing and signing treatment plans, child and adolescent psychiatrists assume responsibility for assessing improvement. Available instruments can be used in quality assurance programs for assessing improvement, monitoring outcome and quality, and at times determining the appropriate level of care. For example, the Child and Adolescent Functional Assessment Scale (Hodges 1994) can be used to help determine a child's eligibility for different levels of service, monitor functional improvement over time, and determine whether services have been utilized appropriately for the needs of each child. With their knowledge of assessment methods and their interests in conjunction with other mental health professionals, child and adolescent psychiatrists can aid agencies in developing a system to meet the agency's particular needs.

Consulting child and adolescent psychiatrists in rural settings who discover that time is at a premium may conduct "staffings" to maximize their exposure to clinical cases:

> During a CMHC staffing, it was learned that several children who were being seen at monthly intervals had been in outpatient treatment for 6 months. Their Child Behavior Checklist (Achenbach 1991) scores were presented and compared to the baseline profiles measured at admission. When total scores were found that demonstrated no clinically significant change, discussions were held with the clinicians about frequency of therapy, goals of therapy, and measurement of change at more frequent intervals to monitor clinical status and response to treatment.

Practice in Community Settings

Community situations needing the help of child and adolescent psychiatrists are abundant. Clinical practice affords opportunities to serve as diagnostician, evaluator, psychopharmacologist, interdisciplinary collaborator, reviewer and supervisor, and individual and family therapist. Community child and adolescent psychiatrists often join interdisciplinary teams of mental health professionals who together assume responsibility for components of the care of a youth and his or her family. The agency-based team may include an intake specialist, a primary clinician, a case manager, a nurse specialist, and a child and adolescent psychiatrist. Primary clinicians may be social workers, licensed counselors, nurses, or psychologists. For severely emotionally disturbed youths, the team may include behavior specialists, intensive case managers, therapeutic support staff to provide wraparound services, and early childhood or general educational specialists. Because of the many community roles available to them, it is imperative that all child and adolescent psychiatrists have a clear definition of the psychiatric role as well as the roles of other team members. Regular team meetings facilitate professional dialogue and subsequent role clarification. Adequate time for communication is a prerequisite for team effectiveness. Psychiatrists, particularly part-time employees within an agency, often appear elusive. Team meetings can help personalize these clinicians and demystify their role.

The child and adolescent psychiatrist functioning as a member of a multidisciplinary behavioral health team faces unique challenges and requires specific skills. To meet these contemporary challenges, training programs emphasize a variety of skills, including eclectic theoretical orientation, diagnostic skills in applying evidence-based treatment, functional assessment skills, psychopharmacology, treatment planning skills, multidisciplinary team collaboration skills, consultative skills, outcome evaluation skills, case management skills, and child advocacy skills. Successful acquisition of such skills means that the psychiatrist is comfortable with alternative approaches, understands how to meet family needs and expectations, can conduct intelligent dialogue with managed care agencies as a child and family advocate, and is facile with multimodal interventions, including the roles of other agencies and community supports.

When an intake specialist gathers psychosocial and historical data and a nurse or psychologist conducts the biological data collection and mental status examination, the child and adolescent psychiatrist may be asked to review the mutually configured treatment plan or to see the identified client for possible pharmacotherapy. Child and adolescent psychiatrists providing collaborative assessment for managing medication often rely on data gathered by other team members. In these situations, the psychiatrist must review all previously collected data, independently review the symptoms, assess the patient's mental status, and review a summary of previously gathered information with the patient and his or her family.

Intercurrent visits for medication monitoring may be conducted jointly with nurse team collaborators. Psychiatrists assume responsibility for data—including clinical symptoms, improvement, side effects, and vital signs—gathered by any or all team members when cosigning clinical notes or basing the prescribing of medication on this information. The provision of service has moved to a collaborative community behavioral health care model that can be more efficient and broad in its scope. Physicians who assume ultimate responsibility for patient care must depend on and trust their collaborators and the information elicited in the sometimes cumbersome process.

Although the approach requires more collaborative efforts with team members, some child and adolescent psychiatrists working in the public sector see youngsters and families for evaluation, medication management, or therapeutic treatment in private office settings. The remaining care is typically provided through an agency. On occasion, a consortium of independent practitioners provides components of care, but this approach becomes cumbersome for families, who must travel to several sites to obtain care. Mutual communication of clinical information, progress, and impediments to care then is essential.

In addition to clinical practice, child and adolescent psychiatrists serve in administrative roles in community agencies. These roles include functioning as the interdisciplinary team leader for smooth interdisciplinary coordination of care, overseeing clinical practice development in an agency or across sites (e.g., managed care contracting), providing oversight of utilization review and quality improvement activities, broad program and infrastructure development, and oversight of outcome measurement and tracking. Child and adolescent psychiatrists who are involved in issues associated with staff productivity or quality of care must be cautious. When misapplied, quality improvement techniques can become punitive. To avoid being viewed as agents for managers who are seeking to discipline the clinical staff, child and adolescent psychiatrists need to know how quality improvement data will be utilized. Often simply explaining the issues and risks to an open-minded administrator can elicit enough understanding to permit modifications to be made that will allow the process to continue positively. The following vignette illustrates a collaborative approach:

> Working on behalf of a school, a child and adolescent psychiatrist was asked to evaluate a 6-year-old boy. Born cocaine exposed and premature, the boy was taken into foster care immediately after birth. After 3 years he was reunited with his mother, who was eager to care for him. The boy's mother had schizoaffective disorder and comorbid substance abuse. During subsequent exacerbations of both disorders in the mother, the boy was cared for by a maternal aunt, who requested help for her nephew's long-standing difficulty with inattention, impulsivity, and hyperactivity that impaired his functioning at home and at school. He had begun threatening his younger siblings, wetting his bed, and playing with matches. His mother had recently completed long-term treatment in a partial hospitalization program. After extensive discussion with the family's physician, a school social worker, and a guidance counselor—along with review of academic, medical, and social service records and an evaluative session with the boy and his aunt and mother—the child and adolescent psychiatrist completed the evaluation. The child was diagnosed with attention-deficit/hyperactivity disorder and acute stress disorder after disclosure of recent sexual abuse by a neighbor friend.
>
> In the biopsychosocial formulation, the child and adolescent psychiatrist addressed the heritable vulnerability to thought, mood, and substance abuse disorders and noted the child's prenatal exposure to cocaine as a possible contributor to the neurobiological diathesis of his attention-deficit/hyperactivity disorder. The aunt was found to be remarkably competent, and the mother demonstrated a desire to have a caring and viable relationship with her son. The boy was found to have an engaging nature and competent social skills along with significant distractibility and hyperactivity. The child articulated worry about his mother's illness and welfare and that he might be "too much for her to handle," while expressing fear and shame about the recent episode of sexual abuse.

The child and adolescent psychiatrist can assist in the family's care in several ways. Having completed the biopsychosocial assessment, the child and adolescent psychiatrist may meet with other interdisciplinary team members to define a treatment plan and address biopsychosocial interventions. Roles might include leading the team, chairing the discussion, and signing off on the treatment plan as the physician of record. The child and adolescent psychiatrist may also provide psychopharmacological management, participate in treatment plan reviews and updates at regular intervals, and provide collaborative guidance to other team members as requested (e.g., suggestions about strategic therapeutic interventions or clarification of medication response or side effects). In some settings, another member of the interdisciplinary team serves as coordinator of team meetings and treatment planning conferences.

The Child and Adolescent Psychiatrist's Signature of Medical Record

A child and adolescent psychiatrist's signature on a medical or clinical record implies that he or she 1) has had direct patient contact, 2) prepared the document unless otherwise specified, and 3) takes responsibility for the content of the record.

Consultation to Community Agencies

The task at hand for the child and adolescent psychiatrist in the role of consultant is that of providing technical advice rather than serving as a clinical or administrative practitioner. Consultants are invited guests offering input to colleagues who have expertise in their own right. The advice provided to those clients or systems should improve the consultee's competence or effectiveness. The consultant's challenge is to join with the clinician, clinical team, or organization in an effort to appreciate the question asked, to know and respect the culture of the agency, to understand the hierarchy of its leadership, and to proceed with data gathering while maintaining respect for the consultee, client, and organization and also developing relevant, concise recommendations that will be easy to implement. The following case example illustrates some of these challenges:

> A child and adolescent psychiatrist provided consultation to a residential adolescent substance abuse program. During a clinical case review, concerns were noted about a very irritable youth who was noncompliant with the treatment program. The psychiatrist raised the possibility that the adolescent was depressed and could benefit from an antidepressant. Staff members expressed concern about labeling the client and using a drug to treat a substance-abusing client. The psychiatrist was placed on the defensive.

In this example, the staff, who come from a different theoretical perspective, have challenged the psychiatrist and have possibly diminished the impact of the consultation. Recognizing the limitations of psychiatric consultation at this time, the psychiatrist may be able to set more modest immediate goals. The psychiatrist has now learned the need for staff education and can initiate discussions with the program's administrator about beginning in-service education and training. The child and adolescent psychiatrist is aware that a consultative relationship should begin with a clear plan and contract and understands the need to work directly with the agency administrator, who provides the mandate for the consultative relationship through developing an agreement with the person empowered to carry out the consultation. The principles of entering and conducting consultation are more fully described in Chapter 1, "Working Within Communities."

Given the initial experience described above, the psychiatrist may consult to this agency in many possible ways. Much depends on how the scope of consultative services to the agency is defined. Because the task is to elucidate the approach to key questions for the consultee, the consultant should alert all parties that information provided might not be kept confidential if the psychiatrist were to answer a question for a third party (e.g., a forensic psychiatrist working for the court must make it clear that interview information will be shared with the court). Similarly, a consulting psychiatrist may be working for an administrator to improve a clinical system. Rather than choose a path that precludes maintaining confidentiality, the psychiatrist may prefer to approach the consultation in a manner that enables the consultee to facilitate change; the consultant can thereby avoid simply reporting to administrators what agency personnel have stated. Occasionally, while serving as the invited guest and consultant, the child and adolescent psychiatrist may meet resistance from staff members or the agency as a whole. As a specialist in behavioral health, the psychiatrist's task is to embrace the resistance as a form of communication. Does it mean that conflicting expectations exist? Could there be poor communication about a new process? Are staff not ready to make an institutional change that has been implemented? With ever-increasing pressures for all agencies to be fiscally solvent and with less funding available, pressures to taper services may be universally applied. The consultant may uncover ethical dilemmas within the institution or among the staff. The job is to define the problem and the available options while continuing to advocate for the best possible care for the youngsters and their families. When the consultation is complete, it is important to summarize the findings and recommendations in a concise and user-friendly fashion. Suggestions should be concrete and feasible (proposing that, e.g., a child and family should be seen at the agency four times weekly when compliance is a problem and agency staff are overextended will not serve the youth or the agency well) and should be contained in a short written report available for review. Detailing critical issues, convening a conference to help the staff brainstorm and develop a workable plan that will be effective, defining clinical problems, offering practical solutions, and presenting findings to the team charged with the task of making it happen are likely to result in a successful consultation termination.

Although consultation can be a rewarding professional activity, there are several pitfalls that child and adolescent psychiatrists should strive to avoid.

Consultants are expected to help with defining the options and the likely outcomes or consequences of each potential choice; however, consultants should never become so personally invested in the outcome for an agency or a family that they feel compelled to insist that recommendations be accepted. They need to be cautious not to overstep their role and take over and not to get drawn into organizational politics. Finding a way to understand the difficulty as it might affect the agency's functioning, without taking sides or offering unsolicited potential solutions, is the ideal.

Typical CMHC Clinical Model

The typical interdisciplinary model for a child and adolescent psychiatrist employed within a CMHC is outlined below:

- The child and adolescent psychiatrist provides psychiatric evaluation of patients and consultation to CMHC clinical team members.
- A social worker or counselor provides psychotherapy.
- A nurse provides psychoeducation and participates in medication management.
- A psychologist administers psychological testing.
- A case manager provides linkage to psychiatric, medical, and community services.

▌ FUNDING THE SERVICES OF THE CHILD AND ADOLESCENT PSYCHIATRIST

It is essential to understand how child and adolescent psychiatric services can be funded. Community psychiatrists providing clinical services have traditionally been funded on a fee-for-service basis, as salaried employees of a community mental health or other agency, or as independent contractors. Those providing care in private practice settings to public-sector patients have billed for their services and have received a rate determined by state Medicaid regulations. Sometimes the rules interfere with best practices. Until recently in North Carolina, billing for pharmacological management was limited to one visit per month. Such rules encourage the private sector to relegate care of Medicaid patients to publicly funded agencies. Some practitioners choose to use alternative billing codes that allow visits at more frequent intervals. Child and adolescent psychiatrists need to be aware of the codes being submitted under their names and also need to be sure that the chart supports the use of those codes.

In the complex world of privatization, child and adolescent psychiatrists may find themselves working for agencies and companies that can be nonprofit or for profit. Unlike community mental health centers, these agencies may not have a full array of services, necessitating communication with multiple other agencies employing case managers or therapists. Furthermore, the administrators of these service-providing agencies may expect high volume case loads to offset salaries and no-shows, which do not generate reimbursement. The child and adolescent psychiatrist will need to discuss these concerns with the administration and to draw on resources such as the American Academy of Child and Adolescent Psychiatry to maintain standards of care.

Since states have been given the opportunity to obtain waivers from the Health Care Financing Administration through the Social Security Act (under sections 1915(b) [Social Security Act, 42 USC 1396n] and 1112 [Social Security Act, 42 USC 1312]), states have been able to use Medicaid funds to develop managed care funding systems. In some states, fee-for-service has been replaced by a reimbursement rate for medically necessary services or by a capitated rate for behavioral health care provided to a population of individuals. The individual practitioner can receive a managed fee as a network clinical care provider but is poorly positioned to participate in capitated plans. Capitated plans are designed so that behavioral health care systems can deliver all components of care in a cost-effective and efficient manner. Child and adolescent psychiatrists working in capitated systems of care will likely participate as independent contractors or employed physicians. In independent contracting arrangements, child and adolescent psychiatrists charge a fee to provide service to an agency. They receive no support for clinical operations beyond the contracted fee-for-service and assume responsibility for the costs of maintaining their practice, including office rent, staffing costs, liability coverage, and other expenses. The paying agency bills the managed care company for the physician's services and keeps the reimbursement.

As an agency employee, the child and adolescent psychiatrist receives a salary, benefits, professional liability coverage, office space, and other support as negotiated. The child and adolescent psychiatrist's services are billed by the agency, and the agency retains the reimbursement.

Child and adolescent psychiatrists serving as consultants are in a more complicated funding position. When conducting evaluations in the service of addressing specific clinical consultation questions, these services are billable. Other consultative services are helpful to an organization's functioning but are not typically billable services. The agency requesting services ideally has funding sources for such activities or may account for them as business expenses.

Most child and adolescent psychiatrists functioning as administrators are full-time employees and are often perceived as expensive. Increasingly, business administrators' salaries are competitive with physicians' incomes, and this bodes well for the child psychiatric administrator. As with any administrative position, the institution must value the training and background of the administrator and must know that this skill set improves the agency's fiscal bottom line. With the increased penetration of capitated reimbursement, the child and adolescent psychiatrist can make critical clinical decisions, assist in the development of care paths, and configure an integrated system of delivery of care that allows patients to make transitions through levels of care in a clinically and fiscally sound fashion.

When configuring a contract for employment, consultation, or independent work, it is essential for child and adolescent psychiatrists to clearly define their responsibilities and those of the other party. All contracts should be clearly delineated and signed before services are provided. Employment contracts include definitions of salary and benefits, which typically include health insurance, professional liability insurance, disability insurance, leave and conference time, and allocation for professional dues and travel expenses. Employed physicians usually have productivity expectations and productivity reviews at regular intervals, often annually.

Child and adolescent psychiatrists who maintain an office-based practice can choose to provide care through contracts with third-party payers on a fee-for-service or a capitated basis. This requires signing a contract to be an in-network provider with an insurance company or managed care organization. It is important to ensure that the fees or capitated rate will allow completion of the clinical work necessary while still covering office expenses. Contracts should not include "hold harmless" clauses that release third-party payers of their liability responsibility. Such a clause may invalidate professional liability coverage. It is essential to review specific contract terms and perhaps even review questions and concerns with an attorney before signing. The American Academy of Child and Adolescent Psychiatry is also developing policies and guidelines for managed care contracts as an aid for its members. The following are prototypical models depicting such funding:

- Employed full- or part-time
- Independent contracting
- Private practice with fee-for-service through payment out-of-pocket, insurance reimbursement, or managed care

▌ CONCLUSIONS

The child and adolescent psychiatrist has the training and experience to function in a wide range of clinical and professional roles within community settings. Clinical work can take place in varied professional settings and through various funding arrangements to ensure optimal use of skills. Community practices allow the child and adolescent psychiatrist a multitude of opportunities to remain active, dynamic, and creative and to provide high-quality mental health care.

❙ REFERENCES

Achenbach TM: Manual for the Child Behavior Checklist/4–18 and 1991 Profile. Burlington, University of Vermont, Department of Psychiatry, 1991

American Academy of Child and Adolescent Psychiatry: Guidelines Regarding the Use of Psychiatrists' Signatures. Washington, DC, American Academy of Child and Adolescent Psychiatry, 1996

Hodges K: Child and Adolescent Functional Assessment Scale. Ypsilanti, Eastern Michigan University, Department of Psychology, 1994

Social Security Act, 42 USC 1312

Social Security Act, 42 USC 1396n

Stroul BA, Friedman RM: A System of Care for Children and Youth With Severe Emotional Disturbances. Washington, DC, Georgetown University Child Development Center, CASSP Technical Assistance Center, 1986

6 ROLE OF THE CLINICAL CHILD PSYCHOLOGIST

Lawrence A. Vitulano, Ph.D.

John R. Holmberg, Psy.D.

In the modern mental health services world, psychiatrists, psychologists, social workers, and the cadre of other mental health care providers have united as collaborators in the movement of contemporary treatment from independent, individual-focused treatment centers to coordinated, community-based programs capable of providing a wide range of interventions and treatment services. Collaboration between mental health care providers, who traditionally had very clear and distinct roles, has allowed for a heightened sharing of knowledge, skill, and talent. In this chapter, we describe qualifications of psychologists, illustrate the history and training of psychology practice, and explore the roles and functions that psychologists offer to community programs.

■ QUALIFICATIONS OF PSYCHOLOGISTS AND WHAT IS UNIQUE ABOUT WHAT THEY DO

Clinical psychologists have followed a prescribed pathway of graduate course work and clinical experiences—based on a history of scientific inquiry—that qualify them to adopt the title of psychologist. Although many care providers take various courses in psychology, only doctoral-level psychologists who have completed an internship can be licensed to work independently as psychologists providing clinical and consultation services in the community. School psychologists constitute an exception; they may obtain certification to work independently within schools and related areas with their specialized master's degree. Historically, psychology emerged as a science in the late 1800s, primarily within university laboratories in Europe and America. By the end of World War II, grand strides had been taken toward creating an integrated paradigm of clinical research and broadly focused intervention strategies. The scientist-practitioner degree in psychology (also known as the Boulder model for training) was established during the landmark 1949 American Psychological Association and U.S. Public Health Service conference held in Boulder, Colorado, to standardize graduate training in clinical psychology. Training in this scientist-practitioner tradition continues today as the guiding philosophy in psychology. Clinical psychology training programs accredited by the American Psychological Association currently allow scientist-practitioners to specialize their craft to some degree, although they still maintain curricula in the core knowledge areas necessary for psychologists who must fill many roles throughout contemporary medical and mental health care.

From the beginning of the twentieth century until the 1949 Boulder conference, psychology had not yet strayed far from research laboratories and consulting rooms housed throughout the military and in outpatient clinics and universities. In the 1960s, psychologists began to assert and extend their skill and expertise to reach those in need in the community. While expanding into a range of community interventions, psychology also had an important influence on the civil rights movement, the Community Mental Health Centers Act of 1963 (P.L. 88-164), and innovative national developmental initiatives such as Head Start.

Although many leaders of psychology are well known to psychiatrists and other mental health professionals, Seymour Sarason is known today primarily among community-focused psychologists (Reppucci 1990; Sarason 1988). During the 1960s, Sarason started one of the first community-based intervention programs, through which he promoted the philosophy that effective services would have to be more readily available to all people and that people should target problems within the communities in which they live. Based on the ideas of Sarason and others, the theoretical interaction between individuals, families, and natural groups within communities set the stage for many of the ecological and systemic theories that guide and inspire community programs today. The movement of psychology from clinics into the community ultimately resulted in the development of a specialized degree in community psychology. At the 1965 Swampscott conference in Massachusetts, it was established that community psychologists would reflect a specialization that focuses on intervention and impetus for change at community and socio-political levels rather than on individuals within communities (Duffy and Wong 1996).

Today most intervention programs employ psychologists whose training as scientist-practitioners prepares them to provide a wide range of professional functions. A unifying criterion for clinical psychologists is that all have attained a doctoral degree from an advanced college, university, or professional school. Three training tracks exist within clinical psychology that allow for a degree of specialization in the field. The first track, providing emphasis on research and teaching, results in the doctor of philosophy (Ph.D.) degree. The second track provides emphasis on clinical interventions and results in the doctor of psychology (Psy.D.) degree. Finally, psychologists who come from programs in the school of education receive a doctor of education (Ed.D.) degree.

Despite the relative differences, all clinical graduate programs provide training in each of the following areas: 1) research methodology, design, and execution; 2) assessment, testing, and evaluation; 3) intervention and therapy; 4) teaching and supervision; 5) consultation and program evaluation; 6) administration and management; and 7) grant solicitation and writing. Along with didactic instruction, observing clinicians in action and doing supervised work are also important aspects of a psychologist's training. Most clinical programs offer hands-on practicum experiences during several years of the academic portion of psychologist training. Today, many if not most of these experiences are in community-based programs. After completing the didactic, practical, and research training, clinical psychologists then complete a year of full-time internship followed by 1 or more years of supervised post-doctoral training before becoming licensed.

In addition to clinical psychologists, many other mental health professionals from a wide range of backgrounds intervene with psychological methods in community-based programs. Specialists in areas such as developmental psychology, industrial and organizational psychology, marital and family counseling, social work, school psychology (from education programs), drug and alcohol counseling, nursing, and rehabilitation use psychological principles to provide valued interventions in community-based programs.

With an understanding of how psychologists are trained, we can turn to the wide range of professional adaptive skills that have helped the field of psychology maintain itself as an invaluable and unique contributor in providing modern mental health services. Contemporary psychology represents the current manifestation of a long evolution in the science of psychology, and, unsurprisingly, its practitioners are attempting to facilitate change in a range of social venues. Today, psychologists are fulfilling professionally diverse roles in community-oriented intervention programs for a range of organizations, such as social service agencies, public and private schools, juvenile justice and detention agencies, and community mental health centers, as well as participating in in-home interventions and prevention and outreach programs.

Psychology, psychiatry, and the other mental health care fields have all undoubtedly been nourished by the same plentiful source of knowledge, which was mapped by trailblazers such as Breuer, Freud, Jung, Kraepelin, and Skinner and by battalions of talented clinicians and theoreticians who followed. Still, since the 1900s, clinical psychology has made unique contributions to modern mental health care and continues to influence many community interventions.

∎ ROLE OF COMMUNITY CHILD PSYCHOLOGISTS

Psychologists practicing in community settings have multiple roles and functions:

- *Research:* Design and execution
- *Assessment:* Observation and testing
- *Intervention:* Psychotherapy and behavior therapy
- *Training:* Teaching and supervision
- *Administration:* Agency and program
- *Consultation:* Individual and program
- *Grant writing:* Clinical research and program support

Research

Research design and execution, one of the first roles for psychologists, remains a core role in community programs. Design and execution of classic research related to human normality and pathology and to effective efforts to alleviate human suffering remain a distinguishing area of expertise for many psychologists. The advent of managed care and the push toward standardization of evidence-based treatment approaches have also led to a boom in community-based programs' outcome research. Given that most treatments conducted in "efficacy" research (i.e., treatment research done by laboratories under strict controls in medical and university clinics) seem to be distant cousins to interventions in community-based programs, it is not immediately evident how traditional outcome research relates to community interventions. Nevertheless, many programs are experiencing increasing demands from financial managers and funding providers to demonstrate accountability and positive effectiveness (i.e., real-world) results; because of these demands, research has been wedged into community-based work. In the near future, even community programs with long histories and impeccable reputations will be applying sound research methods to capture and summarize the impacts of their interventions.

A psychologist's background in research using efficient and simple but change-sensitive evaluation measures will prove invaluable to community programs researching their outcomes. Evaluating outcomes may not seem to be a difficult task, but one must consider the overabundance of factors inherent in community-based work that can create sufficient statistical noise to overshadow a program's positive impact on an individual, family, or community. To ensure that a community program can sufficiently demonstrate effectiveness and justify future funding, measurement of outcomes has to be integrated into the culture and philosophy of the program. The measures a program chooses to use may be as important as other factors such as the building's location and staff diversity. How team leaders and administrators present and monitor the collection of research measures and materials to busy clinicians is also important. If current measures do not demonstrate the changes that the program facilitates, then creating and validating measures is essential to ongoing clinical work. Once the importance and usefulness of standardized measures become part of the treatment culture, outcomes can speak boldly and clearly about the program's impact. Several compendiums (e.g., Maruish 1999; Sederer and Dickey 1996) include descriptions of the basics of outcome measurement and some of the commonly used statistically sensitive measures that are appropriate for use in outcome assessment and quality assurance programs.

Assessment, Testing, and Evaluation

Psychological testing has grown and evolved considerably from the early statistical and measurement principles developed by Galton, Wundt, Binet, and Cattell. Contemporary psychologists are carefully trained to administer standardized and validated measures for testing and assessing individuals in each of the major domains of overall functioning. The domains most frequently assessed in children include current level of development or age equivalent; intelligence and cognitive functioning across a variety of processing abilities; academic achievement; personality, coping, and defensive strategies; type and severity of psychopathology; neuropsychological dysfunction; and acquisition of adaptive or independence skills. Having a wide range of assessment measures allows psychologists to tailor a short battery of tests that can "partial out" or pinpoint answers to complex, interrelated questions about a child's or adolescent's diagnosis, inner life (e.g., thoughts, beliefs, attributions, emotional functioning, heuristics for approaching the world, and coping and defensive strategies), and overall functioning that would otherwise have to be gradually evaluated by clinicians working in the community. One must remember that even seasoned clinicians can be misled into making unreliable estimates of psychological functioning based on interview or observational data alone. Without proper psychological evaluation, cognitively impaired children are often misdiagnosed as having conduct disorders, and children with learning disabilities are often misdiagnosed as being depressed. Psychological testing can be valuable in community-based work.

Intervention

Intervention continues to provide an important role for psychologists, although community-based interventions are an increasingly important focus of attention. Treatment approaches developed and researched by psychologists over the years, both independently and in collaboration with psychiatrists and social workers, have undoubtedly had a significant impact on modern mental health care. In addition to the wealth of knowledge from the psychoanalytic tradition, important historical contributions include the findings of applied behaviorists such as John Watson and B.F. Skinner and the interpersonal approaches developed and described by Carl Rogers and others.

To stay current with the rapidly changing field of mental health services, contemporary training for psychologists continues to evolve and adapt. Besides training in intervention strategies in the community, psychologists now receive specialized training in the use of empirically validated treatment techniques; the use and adaptation of standardized or manualized treatments; and ways to provide sound, focused, brief treatment within the fiscal constraints of managed care. Integration of guiding psychosocial theories (i.e., cognitive-behavioral, psychoanalytic/dynamic, developmental, family systems, and interpersonal), whether by technical or theoretical integration, is an important component in most contemporary training programs. Increased emphasis on collaboration and consultation with medical providers has also emerged as an important training goal for psychology. Along with academic training in neuroanatomy, neuropharmacology, and psychoneuroimmunology that provides psychologists with necessary base knowledge, training in the coordination of treatment providers for continuity and integration of care has also become important in today's psychology training programs.

Teaching, Training, Supervision, and Administration

Teaching, training, supervision, and administration are also roles that psychologists often fill in community-based programs. There is significant overlap in these functions, particularly between supervision and administration (see Chapter 1, "Working Within Communities"). Today there is rich cross-hybridization of supervisors in many community-based programs, in which young clinicians from one discipline will have a senior supervisor from another discipline. Mental health professionals are familiar with traditional teaching methods such as seminars, lectures, observation, and supervision (either individual or group), all of which continue to have their place in community-based work. Directors of community programs often find that these traditional teaching methods have to be extended and adapted in terms of both process and content to fit their clinicians' needs.

The need for flexibility and immediacy in community-based work often requires that supervisors be available on an as-needed basis around the clock. Crises in the community frequently occur outside the working hours of the clinic and demand rapid response from the providers involved. In many programs, this need is accommodated by design, with clinicians being available on a rotating 24-hour call, but often with little immediate supervision of such work. When exceptionally complex or distressing issues arise, even experienced clinicians can feel unsupported, lost, and in crisis themselves—instead of promoting a sense of coherence and crisis de-escalation for the child and family. Although emergency supervision is not foreign to medical providers based in hospital settings, in community-based programs the need to schedule rotations for emergency consultation and clinical backup is often learned through trial and error.

On-call rotation supervisors should know the nature of the work well and be familiar with the patient population. Of course, it is best if supervisors are aware of high-risk patients and their impending treatment issues and plans. Weekly clinical team rounds in which brief clinical updates are recorded have proved to be invaluable in this regard. Rounds also provide a helpful forum for sharing different clinical perspectives about the cases and for brainstorming about available resources and interventions. The richness of collaboration between workers in psychiatry, psychology, social work, and mental health is most evident during team rounds. Each discipline brings unique and shared perspectives, which allow the team to conceptualize a child's difficulties in multiple dimensions. In our experience, team rounds are best viewed as a supplement, not a replacement for individual supervision. Community interventions are often stressful, difficult, and complex; even seasoned clinicians find that engaging in consultation and having time to talk through their interventions with colleagues are essential elements for conducting effective work. Such a supervisory model is most helpful when it becomes part of the collaborative treatment culture rather than a forum related to power or control within the organization. These efforts also promote a program culture grounded in respect and interdisciplinary collaboration that unifies treatment teams who are able to survive the storm of obstacles (e.g., funding, legal, staffing) that inevitably encumber community-based work. Many of these supervisory efforts (e.g., supervising the on-call clinician, holding team rounds) are costly and have little or no basis for reimbursement from third-party payers. To adapt, programs must bundle these costs into the fees or the grant requests that finance the program.

Nevertheless, not all topics are best handled in team rounds or supervision. Collaboratively led seminars also provide a useful forum for teaching and cooperation. Traditional topics such as cognitive-behavioral treatment techniques, research, and theoretical issues are often covered, but the type of work done by community-based programs brings with it inherent difficulties that need to be addressed and revisited through group didactic training (e.g., many programs overlook teaching clinicians about issues such as personal safety and security, although it is a vitally important topic, discussed below).

Administration

Psychologists have served as agency as well as program administrators, and safety illustrates a typical administrative area. It is not self-evident to many traditionally trained clinicians that they must be quite familiar with the neighborhoods that they are entering. Nor is it self-evident that personal safety takes precedence over any therapeutic action. Clinical work cannot be done without a feeling of safety and freedom to give the fullest attention to the patient.

Other program-level actions have proven helpful in addressing safety issues with clinicians. Besides training, community programs will likely need to budget money for multiple-use pagers and emergency cellular phones for field-workers. It can also be helpful to designate someone (e.g., the program administrative assistant) as the home-base contact, with whom clinicians can check in and leave their schedules between visits. Other more specific safety issues (e.g., parking, when to request escorts by police, and safety awareness within patients' homes) also need to be explicitly and directly addressed. Programs often adopt a partner-based approach to community interventions for a variety of reasons, but safety is another good reason to advocate for such an approach.

In addition to dealing with issues of safety in training and supervision, contemporary psychologists have become increasingly aware of and attuned to the ways in which individual differences (i.e., developmental, gender, sexual preference, racial, and cultural) must be integrated into successful interventions, especially in community-based programs (Aguirre 1998). This increased awareness of individual differences has provided for greater diversification within another of the traditional roles for psychologists in the community: consultation and program evaluation.

Consultation and Program Evaluation

For years psychologists have provided consultations to businesses, corporations, and programs to address a range of goals such as improved operations, increased productivity, decreased staff conflicts, and heightened profit margins. Psychology consultations can be quite limited. For example, a program supervisor might request to have the staff surveyed regarding topics of interest for an in-service consultation, which the psychologist then prepares or arranges for a specialist to conduct. In program evaluations, psychologists often conduct a study of organizational functions such as intra-agency communication, responsiveness to crisis situations, or costs and benefits of flextime versus overtime work schedules. Program evaluations can also focus on broader issues such as the demographics of patients served, overlaps or gaps in services provided by the agency and other programs in the community, or the need for additional services in the area (e.g., parent support groups, parent guidance, therapy for parents). Today, in addition to these traditional consultations, many organizations retain psychologists to assess their ability to meet the needs of minority groups within the population served as well as within the organization.

Because most organizations are complex, most program evaluations are equally complex. The many procedures and issues to consider—and the wide scope of review that effective program evaluations use—contribute to this complexity. Common misperceptions abound within each organizational level as to the purpose and utility of a consultation (consultants are generally viewed as outside experts who have been brought to the agency to make sweeping changes and cuts because the staff is not performing adequately). Modern program evaluators try to address these concerns by 1) working to join with and empower persons from each level of the program and from the broader social systems involved, 2) attempting to gain an authentic view from each of the systemic perspectives by actively participating in the operations as a participant-observer, 3) basing observations from a perspective that focuses on a program's strengths and competencies and how these can be enhanced, and 4) helping individuals and programs see that they have the power and control to make positive changes without threatening the work and well-being that have already been established. To accomplish these goals, program evaluators work with all stakeholders, or people who have a role and investment in the program. The broad lens that the program evaluators use will include perspectives from observational boards and regulatory agencies, administration, management, frontline employees, past and present clients, community persons in need but not receiving services, and broad systemic representatives from state and local governments.

Grant Solicitation and Writing

One of the most important aspects of a contemporary community-based program is how to finance the program. Identifying persons in need, finding appropriate staff, and determining a location are all challenging but manageable tasks; however, the difficulty of securing funding to start and then maintain a service for those in need of it—some of whom are unable to pay any amount—often stops a good idea before it can be implemented. Although certain services (e.g., direct clinical contacts) warrant reimbursement by commercial or government-funded insurance, the time-intensive process of obtaining the fees can make the seeking of such funds seem less worthwhile. Many aspects of the ethical and effective provision of mental health services in the community are not reimbursed by payers. A short list includes clinician travel, clinicians being on call without a crisis to respond to, supervision, rounds, paperwork, insurance authorization and billing, research, training, and quality assurance efforts. Even this short list illustrates why it is hard to keep even the tightest-run program afloat. Alternative funding sources are simply a must in community-focused interventions, but those funds tend to be available in cycles rather than from consistent and reliable sources. For all these reasons, bringing a psychologist on board who brings experience in securing research money and who can ferret out grants, work with benevolent associate grantors, and ensure that funding will be available in the long term can be invaluable to community-based programs. Community clinical psychologists can also be helpful in working at sociopolitical levels to gain direct, legislated funds to maintain effective programs.

▌ CONCLUSIONS

Community work by psychologists has its roots in the community mental health movement initiated by the federal government in 1961. Since that time, clinical psychologists have shifted their focus from an individual perspective to a more ecological one, emphasizing empowerment and long-term systemic change. Because community mental heath needs and resources change rapidly, psychologists performing community work must be flexible in the roles they assume. Psychology continues to build on its strong scientific foundations, and the principles of empiricism, learning, and behavior have always guided its practice. Now the challenge is to create innovative programs based on sound scientific foundations to meet the growing needs of diverse communities. To accomplish this task, psychologists must first formulate the right questions to ask—questions that are relevant and testable—to collect the data necessary to evaluate the plethora of new programs that purport to effect long-term systemic change in their communities. Much interest has been drawn to the reallocation of community resources in an attempt to address community problems more efficiently and inexpensively. New collaborations between overlapping service providers have been fostered, and previously helpless groups of individuals have been empowered with the skills necessary to make decisions for themselves and to plan for their future. The pressures of managed care have forced traditional systems to revise their models and provide alternative services to a variety of populations in need of help. Perhaps one of the most advantageous changes in community programs has been the increased access to services through home-based and other outreach programs. Attention to prevention has also risen as programs in the community attend to both systemic and individual targets for community intervention. Because psychology is no longer interested only in an $N{=}1$ model, community psychology has introduced concern for the largest Ns and has thus moved to influencing policy making at a national level. The future promises new, exciting, integrated and collaborative models for the delivery of mental health services in previously underserved communities.

❚ REFERENCES

Aguirre A: Community mental health services in a managed care environment: 10 key issues in promoting cultural competence, in Promoting Cultural Competence in Children's Mental Health Services (Systems of Care for Children's Mental Health Series). Edited by Hernandez M, Isaacs MR. Baltimore, MD, Paul Brookes, 1998, pp 95–115

Community Mental Health Centers Act of 1963, Pub. L. No. 88-164, 77 Stat. 282

Duffy KG, Wong FY: Community Psychology. Boston, MA, Allyn & Bacon, 1996

Maruish ME: The Use of Psychological Testing for Treatment Planning and Outcomes Assessment, 2nd Edition. Mahwah, NJ, Erlbaum, 1999

Reppucci ND: The conscience of community psychology: Seymour Sarason's contributions. Am J Community Psychol 18:353–358, 1990

Sarason SB: The Making of an American Psychologist: An Autobiography. San Francisco, CA, Jossey-Bass, 1988

Sederer LI, Dickey B: Outcomes Assessment in Clinical Practice. Baltimore, MD, Williams & Wilkins, 1996

7 ROLE OF THE CHILD MENTAL HEALTH SOCIAL WORKER

John Ronnau, Ph.D., A.C.S.W.

In this chapter, I describe 1) the role of the social work professional in assisting children with serious emotional disturbance (SED) and their families; and 2) the theoretical framework, values, ethics, helping process, and roles of social work. To provide effective community-based social work for children with SED, one must take into account the essential role that families have in the care of these children. The needs of children with SED are extensive, complex, and long lasting and involve numerous social institutions, including those related to child welfare, law, mental health, education, and medicine (Bruner 1991; Stroul and Friedman 1986). Effective support for families who care for these children requires collaborative work from a variety of professionals.

The family is the most important resource for the care of children with SED. The parent is the one most directly involved in the provision of day-to-day care and the management and coordination of services for the child (Lourie 1995). The parent is typically the one who must get the child to the doctor, to school, to the therapist, and to recreational activities. Although intensive inpatient treatment may at times be needed along with numerous other services, the best predictor of a positive outcome for a child with SED is the presence of a long-term, committed caregiver (J. Ronnau, "Ordinary Families— Extraordinary Care Giving: The Strengths of Families Caring for Children With SED," unpublished data, May 1988). The goal of the professional should be to support, not supplant, the youth's family.

▐ THE SOCIAL WORK PERSPECTIVE

Implications for Community-Based Practice

A dual focus on the person and the environment requires social workers to conduct assessments and assist their clients—whether individuals, families, or groups—with a purposeful awareness of the environment (Germain and Gitterman 1996). Social work is distinct from other helping disciplines by virtue of its "dual focus on person and environment, with the emphasis placed on interactions and transactions between them" (Sheafor et al. 1988, p. 13). For example, the assessment, diagnosis, and treatment of depression must take into account the person's internal experience, barriers, and resources in the environment (family, friends, job, neighborhood). Focusing exclusively on intrapsychic issues would constitute irresponsible practice of social work.

Theoretical Framework

Social workers view the world as if through a wide-angle lens because of their profession's eclectic, interdisciplinary knowledge base that draws heavily on the social and behavioral sciences, particularly sociology, psychology, and anthropology (Hoffman and Sallee 1994). National accreditation standards for social work education include a broad foundation in the liberal arts. Social workers are expected to consider the impacts of history, politics, and economics on individual behavior. Their holistic view makes them attentive to emotional, spiritual, and physical needs. Over time, most social workers develop one or more specialty fields of practice (e.g., juvenile justice, medical social work, substance abuse, aging).

Values and Ethics

Self-determination, informed consent, privacy, and confidentiality are among the ethical obligations of social workers that are especially pertinent to community-based work. Social workers are expected to promote their clients' involvement in decision making and must adhere to a code of ethics and standards set forth by their professional organization, the National Association of Social Workers (NASW), for behavior with clients and colleagues and in practice settings and society. These values and ethics have important implications for the ways that social workers interact with clients and other professionals. Clients' self-determination should be limited only when their "actions or potential actions pose a serious, foreseeable, and imminent risk to themselves or others" (National Association of Social Workers 1996a, p. 37). Informed consent is an important precursor to promoting clients' self-determination. Social workers are mandated to explain the purpose of services, potential risks, limitations, costs, reasonable alternatives, the right to refuse or withdraw consent, and the time frame of the consent (National Association of Social Workers 1996a).

Social Work Roles

Depending on the size and needs of the client system, social workers function in many roles: enabler, facilitator, planner, broker, advocate, convener, mediator, activist, catalyst, teacher, trainer, outreach worker, and researcher (Miley et al. 1995). Some of these roles and services may be billable through third-party insurance funding mechanisms. Managed care plans, for instance, may view them as preventing the use of more intensive and expensive services.

Case Manager Versus Therapist

Two roles often filled by social workers are case manager and therapist. Professional social work requires knowledge and skills inherent in both of these roles. Elements of each are integral to the successful implementation of the other. However, too often they are viewed as incompatible. The roots of case management are in social casework, which has greatly influenced social work (Hamilton 1951; Perlman 1957). Various case management models are used—including those of generalist, specialist, therapist–case manager, and psychosocial rehabilitation center—as well as variations on each of these themes (Rothman 1992). Although there is no universally accepted definition of case manager, under most models the role is diversified and includes multiple tasks and responsibilities, ranging from brokerage of services to advocacy to serving as primary therapist (Rose 1992). The most frequently cited case management functions are needs assessment, service or treatment planning, linking or referring, coordination, outreach, service implementation, monitoring, and advocacy (Rose 1992). These varied, complicated, and demanding functions require the case manager to possess diverse skills and to fulfill a variety of roles. Case managers play a critical role by helping their clients connect with and coordinate needed services.

The role of therapist is often equated with that of clinician. Clinical social workers serve individuals, families, and groups in a variety of public and private nonprofit agencies. The services they provide include prevention, help in coping with current difficulties, stabilization of progress, and remediation of past traumas (Saari 1986). By using their direct knowledge of the client's experience, clinical social workers also work to increase access to social and economic resources. Like other modes of social work, clinical social work makes use of a helping process that includes engagement, assessment and formulation, various types of interventions, and evaluations (Saari 1986). Clinical social workers collaborate with other providers to link and coordinate services and to advocate for their clients.

Administrator

Many social workers eventually take on administrative roles. Although the knowledge base and values of social work are assets, they may further complicate the challenge of administration. Added to the supervisory and educational responsibilities of administrators is an expressive-supportive leadership function. The social work supervisor is expected to sustain worker morale and to respond to job-related discouragement and discontent (Kadushin 1976). Rapp and Poertner (1992) suggested that administrators should promote a "client-centered" approach, keeping the client center stage in the helping process while being attentive to worker satisfaction. Social work administrators may feel caught between agency demands for increased productivity and the emotional needs of workers with excessive case loads. They may feel torn between what their clinical knowledge and experience tell them is best for clients (e.g., more frequent sessions, home-based rather than office contacts) and the limits of care imposed by funding sources.

Consultant

Social workers are especially well suited for the consultant role because in their social work training they have been taught to "start where the client is," to be culturally competent, to use a strength-based approach, to attend to group dynamics, and to work across social systems. Consultation is both a method and a process for disseminating expert knowledge that can improve services for at-risk populations (Rieman 1992). The social worker as consultant serves as facilitator, educator, trainer, and researcher.

Social Work Credentials

A credential signifies that a practitioner has met minimum standards to provide services to the public. Social work is regulated by licensure, certification, or registration in all 50 states, the District of Columbia, and territories. Most states establish regulatory boards to issue licenses to social workers at several levels. The licensed baccalaureate social worker (LBSW) and licensed master social worker (LMSW) credentials indicate completion of an undergraduate or graduate degree at an accredited social work program. Earning certification as a licensed clinical social worker (LCSW) requires specializing in a clinical social work field of study, completing a minimum amount (usually 2 years) of post–master's degree supervised clinical experience, passing a credentialing examination, and earning continuing education credits.

The NASW has developed a system of voluntary certifications. The Academy of Certified Social Workers (ACSW) credential entails 2 years of full-time paid post-master's or postdoctoral social work experience with supervision by an experienced social worker. The qualified clinical social worker (QCSW) credential requires supervision by a clinical social worker and at least 2 years of experience. The diplomate in clinical social work (DCSW) certification entails 3 additional years of full-time clinical social work practice, including 2 years of full-time practice within the past 10 years. The first field-specific credential to be offered by the NASW is certified school social work specialist (C-SSWS), which requires at least 2 years of postgraduate supervised school social work experience. In addition to the requirements already mentioned, each certification requires a master's degree or doctorate in social work from a school accredited by the Council on Social Work Education (CSWE), application and renewal fees, and examinations (QCSW excepted). Certification applicants must agree in writing to practice according to the NASW code of ethics and practice standards and to submit to adjudication proceedings if charged with violations (National Association of Social Workers 1996a, 1996b).

Some states allow for voluntary registration laws and statutory certification in addition to licensing. Social workers are prohibited from using titles (e.g., registered clinical social worker) unless they have been credentialed to do so. Credentialed social workers who violate professional standards are subject to disciplinary actions, including revocation of the license, suspension of the license, probation, a requirement to practice under supervision for a specified period, a fine, or the requirement that the social worker undergo mental health or substance abuse treatment (Biggerstaff 1995).

The Helping Process

The business of social work is to help systems change in positive ways. Change is accomplished through a helping process that is systematic but not linear and that consists of several steps: relationship building, data collection, assessment, planning, implementation, transition, and evaluation (Hoffman and Sallee 1994). The steps are discussed in the subsections that follow, along with some implications for community-based social work.

Relationship Building

The relationship that develops between the client and the social worker is critical to determining the effectiveness of the helping process (Miley et al. 1995). The best way to establish a productive working relationship may be to meet practical needs first; if a family is low on food, their utility bills are past due, or the parents just need a break, it will be difficult for them to engage in therapy until these needs are met.

Data Collection

Data collection is ongoing and begins with the first step in the helping process. Throughout the time a social worker is involved with a family, their biopsychosocial story should be continually updated. New needs will surface and known ones will become better defined. New goals will emerge as others are met or are found to be unrealistic. For instance, teachers, counselors, or probation officers who work with the youth and the family may provide new information that can help the social worker better meet the family's goals. Tools such as genograms, ecomaps, strength-based inventories, problem checklists, and family history questionnaires can be valuable both for information gathering and for furthering therapeutic goals.

Assessment

The most critical step in the social work helping process is assessment. Collecting large amounts of information will not benefit the client unless it is put to good use. Assessment entails sorting, organizing, and prioritizing and must include analysis of the problem, the person, and the ecological context (Hepworth and Larson 1993). Student social workers may assume that intervention steps (e.g., making contracts with clients, engaging in therapy, setting goals) should come first. But these steps may be ineffective or even harmful unless they are preceded by an accurate and thorough assessment based on a comprehensive and accurate data set about the person in the environment.

Planning

An effective plan identifies goals and steps to achieve them, including who will do what and by when. Worker and client responsibilities are clearly spelled out, and goals must clearly pertain to needs identified by the client. The plan must be realistic and achievable and should be revised as needed to reflect the client's changing situation. The best of plans will fail unless the client feels a sense of ownership. In working with families with SED, for instance, it is essential for the social worker to refrain from blaming the parents for the child's problems. Parents of children with SED report that workers who project a judgmental attitude create an impediment to working effectively with them (Ronnau 1989).

Implementation

Once goals have been formulated, steps identified, and responsibilities clarified, the plan is put into action. The action taken is determined by the goals. Social workers must take care to empower their clients, especially during the implementation step of the helping process. One measure of empowerment is whether the client is stronger (more knowledgeable, skillful, confident, capable) after the social worker has left than when the social worker entered his or her life. Empowerment entails involving resources that naturally occur in the client's environment (e.g., friends, neighbors, family members).

Transition

The manner in which social workers manage transitions is critical. The termination process begins during the first contact between the social worker and the client. At that time, the social worker clarifies his or her roles and purpose, agency sanctions and policies, and limits to confidentiality and states the intended frequency and duration of contacts. As the end of the relationship draws near, the social worker notes milestones. For example, mentioning to the client that they have 2 more weeks to work together is a good way to remind all involved (including the social worker) of the finiteness of the helping process.

Evaluation

Evaluation provides closure and helps social workers assess their overall effectiveness. The social worker may use some or all of the following questions during the evaluation process: What has worked and what has not? Which goals were achieved and which were not? What goals remain to be completed? What were some especially helpful things the social worker did? What was not helpful? Also, all of the other professionals involved with the client system should be asked to give their assessment and clarify their future involvement with the family. This step may also involve referrals and linkage to additional services.

Practicing a Strengths Perspective

Use of a strengths perspective is a reemerging trend in social work practice. "The strengths perspective asserts a fundamental premise: that it will be through the mobilization and articulation of inherent talents, abilities, aspirations, resources, wiles and grit that transformation, rebound, and change will occur" (Weick and Saleeby 1995, p. 4). The strengths perspective can be used to find resources within individuals, their families, and their environments to help them solve their problems and reach their goals. Resources are defined very broadly to include talents, skills, knowledge, dreams, and other people (friends, neighbors, extended family). Special attention is paid to past successes. For example, although a parent may be discouraged by one child's school difficulties, another sibling may be doing quite well. Any of these strengths may become resources to solve a problem or meet a need. In the case of one family, an adolescent's dream of becoming a pilot led a social worker to help the family find a neighbor to provide some critical after-school supervision. The neighbor, a mechanic at a small local airport, allowed the youth to look over his shoulder, hand him tools, and help clean up around the shop. The social worker's strengths assessment led to the discovery of this invaluable resource.

Family Involvement

For too long, parents have been blamed for their child's emotional disability and criticized for being too strict or too lenient. If they speak out, they are accused of being overinvolved. If they do not, they are labeled as emotionally distant. They have seldom been treated as partners in the helping process. Their experience as parents of a child with special needs is not valued and is often not solicited. Because they are not perfect parents (none of us are!), their caregiving is considered inferior. Because they are not being paid, their contributions as caregivers are not valued. It should be acknowledged that working 24 hours a day, 7 days a week, all year long at any job presents lots of opportunities to make mistakes—and to do a lot of things right.

Paid professionals will never know the youth as well as the parents do. Parenting children with SED is an exhausting job. As professionals, social workers should support the parent's caregiving role, not supplant it. This stance does not imply that these are perfect parents of perfect families; there are problems, or the family would not be involved in the system. But the family is the expert in many areas—its history, feelings, dreams, culture, and rituals; what has worked with the child and what has not; and what it is like to raise a child who has an SED. If given opportunity and encouragement and treated with genuine respect, parents can be valuable partners in the helping process.

Interdisciplinary Social Work Practice

Social work practice by its very nature is interdisciplinary. The ecological or person-in-environment perspective of social work necessitates that social workers "look holistically at the child, the family, their roots, and their culture" and that they "understand the importance of working with other agencies and delivery systems. Social workers must be skilled both in front line practice with children and families and in working within the larger system" (Zlotnik 1997, pp. 24–25). The necessity for social workers to practice values and skills for maintaining a holistic view, to communicate across organizational boundaries, to facilitate collaborative problem solving, to exchange information, and to build partnerships is well established (Germain and Gitterman 1996; Zlotnik 1997). Hooper-Briar and Lawson (1996) called for the advancement of a "second generation of partnerships" characterized in part by interdisciplinary and interprofessional education and by training and designs that encourage service systems and providers to work interdependently.

Interdisciplinary practice is no shortcut. It is time-consuming and demanding work. But there is no more effective way to assist youths with SED and their families. Their needs are too many and too complex and cut across too many systems to be answered by any one discipline alone. The needs of youths with SED, the families who care for them, and the communities they live in require effective responses from many disciplines to be focused on one common goal: helping these youths become successful adults. Cross-disciplinary work presents many challenges, including turf issues, leadership, status, and information sharing. These challenges can be overcome if each member of the team is respectful toward the others and has a clear understanding of the others' values and theoretical framework. Because of their person-in-environment focus and broad theoretical foundation, social workers are well equipped to be effective team members. The Checklist for Social Workers (see appendix at end of this chapter) provides a useful guide to ensure that the principles of social work are applied within an interdisciplinary context when helping families caring for children with emotional problems.

▌ CONCLUSIONS

Social workers are educated to assess the strengths and needs of families and communities. They can coordinate services and use their clinical skills. They can employ a variety of roles based on the needs of their clients. Their person-in-environment perspective makes them effective interdisciplinary practitioners.

Most families caring for a child with special needs do an admirable job, but they will likely need help from a variety of professionals. Social workers can fill a valuable role as both clinician and coordinator of services in helping these families.

▌ REFERENCES

Biggerstaff MA: Licensing, regulation, and certification, in Encyclopedia of Social Work, 19th Edition. Edited by Beebe L, Winchester NA. New York, National Association of Social Workers, 1995, pp 1616–1624

Bruner C: Thinking Collaboratively: Ten Questions and Answers to Help Policy Makers Improve Children's Services. Washington, DC, Education and Human Services Consortium, 1991

Germain CB, Gitterman A: The Life Model of Social Work Practice, Revised Edition. New York, Columbia University Press, 1996

Hamilton G: Social Casework Theory and Practice. New York, Columbia University Press, 1951

Hepworth DH, Larson JA: Direct Social Work Practice: Theory and Skills, 4th Edition. Belmont, CA, Brooks/Cole, 1993

Hoffman KS, Sallee AL: Social Work Practice: Bridges to Change. Boston, MA, Allyn & Bacon, 1994

Hooper-Briar K, Lawson HA (eds): Expanding Partnerships for Vulnerable Children, Youth, and Families. Alexandria, VA, Council on Social Work Education, 1996

Kadushin A: Supervision Is Social Work. New York, Columbia University Press, 1976

Lourie IS: Foreword, in From Case Management to Service Coordination for Children With Emotional, Behavioral, or Mental Disorders: Building on Family Strengths. Edited by Friesen BJ, Poertner J. Baltimore, MD, Brookes, 1995, pp xiii–xiv

Miley KK, O'Melia M, DuBois B: Generalist Social Work Practice: An Empowering Approach. Boston, MA, Allyn & Bacon, 1995

National Association of Social Workers: Code of Ethics. Washington, DC, National Association of Social Workers, 1996a

National Association of Social Workers: NASW Professional Social Work Credentials. Washington, DC, National Association of Social Workers, 1996b

Perlman HH: Social Casework, a Problem-Solving Process. Chicago, IL, University of Chicago Press, 1957

Rapp CA, Poertner J: Social Administration: A Client-Centered Approach. New York, Longman, 1992

Rieman DW: Strategies in Social Work Consultation. New York, Longman, 1992

Ronnau J: An exploratory multiple-case study of what adolescents with emotional disabilities need to live in the community. Unpublished doctoral dissertation, University of Kansas, Lawrence, KS, 1989

Rose SM: Case Management and Social Work Practice. New York, Longman, 1992

Rothman J: Guidelines for Case Management: Putting Research to Professional Use. Itasca, IL, FE Peacock, 1992

Saari C: Clinical Social Work Treatment: How Does It Work? New York, Gardner, 1986

Sheafor BW, Horejsi CR, Horejsi GA: Techniques and Guidelines for Social Work Practice. Boston, MA, Allyn & Bacon, 1988

Stroul BA, Friedman RM: A System of Care for Severely Emotionally Disturbed Children and Youth. Washington, DC, Georgetown University Child Development Center, CASSP Technical Assistance Center, 1986

Weick A, Saleeby D: A Post Modern Approach to Social Work Practice. Garden City, NY, Adelphi University School of Social Work, 1995

Zlotnik JL: Preparing the Workforce for Family-Centered Practice: Social Work Education and Public Human Services Partnerships. Alexandria, VA, Council on Social Work Education, 1997

APPENDIX
Checklist for Social Workers
Helping Families Caring for Children With Serious Emotional Disturbance

This checklist should be used by the social worker with each family that is caring for a child with a serious emotional disturbance. It serves as a reminder of important steps in the helping process.

1. **As a social worker, I can best help this family by filling the role(s) of (check all that apply)**

    ____enabler ____broker ____mediator ____teacher
    ____facilitator ____advocate ____activist ____trainer
    ____planner ____convener ____catalyst ____researcher
    ____outreach worker

2. **Check each of the steps that have been taken to assist this family:**

    ____relationship building   ____implementation
    ____data collection   ____transition
    ____assessment   ____evaluation
    ____planning

3. **List at least three strengths of each family member:**

    _____
    _____
    _____
    _____

4. **What does each family member say that he or she needs in order to care for the child with serious emotional disturbance?**

    _____
    _____
    _____
    _____

5. List the agencies or systems that need to be involved in helping this family:

_____

_____

_____

_____

8 ROLE OF THE CLINICAL NURSE

Nancy D. Opie, R.N., D.N.S., F.A.A.N.

Brenda L. Costello-Wells, R.N., M.S.N., C.S.

During the 1990s and continuing into the twenty-first century, dramatic changes have occurred in how and where nurses and other health care providers practice and in how their services are funded. As the trend continues toward only brief use of the hospital, greater use of community settings, and increased emphasis on cost containment, the roles of nurses and the settings where they work will continue to change. Like other nurses, child and adolescent psychiatric nurses are struggling to redefine their roles and to acquire the skills and credentials needed for the varied settings and challenges they are confronting. This chapter provides a description of the multiple roles, challenges, and rewards associated with contemporary child and adolescent psychiatric nursing. The role of the advanced practice nurse (APN) is emphasized. Examples of responsibilities associated with prescriptive authority, reimbursement, team membership, and subcontracting to cooperating agencies are provided.

▌ PSYCHIATRIC NURSING PREPARATION

The American Nurses Association (ANA) recognizes three levels of psychiatric nursing practice: nonbaccalaureate, baccalaureate, and master's. The

97

ANA requires applicants to verify their completion of specified amounts of clinical supervision and clinical experience before taking the certification examination. The registered nurse, certified (RN, C) credential designates certification at the nonbaccalaureate level; registered nurse, board certified (RN, BC) designates certification at the baccalaureate level; and advanced practice registered nurse, board certified (APRN, BC) designates certification at the advanced practice level. Because of the requirements of third-party payers, certification is preferred for many community-based programs. In recent years, many nurses have continued their education to obtain a doctoral degree, allowing them to become university faculty members and directors of research and administrative teams.

A master's program requires core studies such as nursing theory and advanced role theory, research methods, and social and political issues related to health delivery systems. In addition, a graduate program in child and adolescent psychiatric nursing includes in-depth study and clinical experiences in the following areas:

- Child and adolescent psychology
- Biopsychosocial and environmental influences on mental health and illness
- Epidemiology of mental illness
- Psychiatric and physical assessment
- Growth and development
- Diagnostic reasoning
- Psychopharmacology
- Theory and techniques of individual, group, and family therapy
- Health promotion and prevention of illness
- Political advocacy
- Community and client partnerships

An APN should also be prepared to collaborate in the research process and to provide mental health consultation. For further information, the reader is referred to Worley 1997.

▌ PRACTICE SETTINGS

Current practice guidelines emphasize providing treatment for children and adolescents in a clinically appropriate situation but in the least restrictive environment possible. Whenever possible, services are provided in community settings to support and maintain the child and family in their home setting. Hospitalization is utilized in critical situations for as brief a period as possible. Thus, mental health professionals must collaborate and contract with community agencies to provide mental health services. Environments for the provision of care in the community include the following:

- Outpatient clinics associated with hospitals
- Community mental health agencies
- Emergency departments
- Primary care settings (clinics and doctors' offices)
- Schools
- Home care agencies
- Day treatment programs
- Runaway shelters
- Shelters for victims of abuse
- Juvenile justice facilities

Therapeutic interventions used by an APN in these settings may include individual therapy, group or family therapy, crisis intervention, and consultation and collaboration with other staff members, such as teachers, administrators, physicians, social workers, home care nurses and aides, and juvenile justice professionals. Prescriptive authority has become a central skill in the role of many APNs. A shortage of child and adolescent psychiatrists and the demand for cost-effective care by consumers and third-party payers have influenced the expansion of this role.

ROLE FUNCTIONS AND RESPONSIBILITIES IN COMMUNITY-BASED CHILD PSYCHIATRIC NURSING

The roles and responsibilities of community-based child and adolescent psychiatric nurses are complex, multifaceted, and challenging. Collaborating and consulting with other professionals and persons involved with child clients are essential. Children and adolescents are not legally responsible for themselves, nor are they independent of parents, guardians, and teachers. Case loads are often replete with crisis-prone families who have limited resources and with children who have multiple problems, such as learning disabilities, anxiety, and depression. Primary physicians are sometimes involved in care as well, and if so they must be consulted. Frequently the caretakers are grandparents or other family members, foster parents, or group home counselors. Therefore, it is essential for community-based child and adolescent psychiatric nurses to have excellent communication skills, cultural competence, a high degree of flexibility, and an open, nonjudgmental attitude.

Table 8-1 provides information on the multiple roles that are commonly available to the APN, and Table 8-2 presents examples of roles available to the registered nurse who is prepared and certified as a generalist psychiatric nurse.

TABLE 8–1.   Roles of an advanced practice nurse

Diagnosing psychiatric disorders

Prescribing medication, under physician supervision

Conducting individual, group, and family therapy

Supervising generalist nurses, nursing students, and other mental health workers

Performing crisis, intake, and triage assessments

Conducting research

Performing administrative tasks

Consulting

Teaching

Performing program development

TABLE 8–2.   Common roles of a generalist child psychiatric nurse

Conducting medication follow-up clinics

Conducting case management

Counseling patients on nutrition and weight management

Directing groups on anger management, stress management, behavior management, and parenting

Maintaining and managing therapeutic environments

Performing client advocacy

Nurses' roles vary based on the client's needs and the agency's purposes and functions. In all roles, the responsibilities of the child and adolescent psychiatric nurse are to promote mental health, prevent mental illness, and prevent sequelae from an episode of mental illness or trauma. In every role, the psychiatric nurse has the duty to protect clients from harming themselves or others, including the duty to warn potential victims of any intended harm. The following case example illustrates some of these roles:

> Mark, a 7-year-old child, was referred to the community mental health center (CMHC) by his school's APN because of bizarre comments he made in the classroom. The child and adolescent APN at the CMHC conducted the initial evaluation and gave Mark a differential diagnosis of "rule out schizophrenia; rule out bipolar disorder; rule out attention-deficit/hyperactivity disorder [ADHD]." At the initial evaluation, Mark was delusional but had no history of hallucinations. He also had extremely rapid cycling of moods, which appeared to his mother and teacher like hyperactivity at times. Because of the complexity of the case, Mark was seen and evaluated by the child psychiatrist, who agreed with the differential diagnosis made by the APN; however, the

psychiatrist was hesitant to diagnose a child of this age with schizophrenia. The primary differential diagnosis was then changed to "rule out psychosis."

After consultation with the child psychiatrist, the APN started Mark on an atypical antipsychotic. The APN planned to stabilize him on this medication and to continue to assess him for ADHD and bipolar disorder. Mark was also evaluated by a child psychologist, who was unable to give a definitive diagnosis. Mark was seen weekly by the APN for medication reviews and for individual therapy focused primarily on assessment and social skills training. His mother received home-based intensive parenting training by a master's-level child therapist. At school, Mark continued to participate in a boys' group focused on social skills and appropriate expression of feelings. He was also selected to participate in Agape, a therapeutic horse-riding program offered at his school, in which he thrived and developed greater self-esteem. The educational team consisted of his teacher, the teacher for emotionally handicapped children, the vice principal, the school nurse, the school-based APN, Mark, and his mother. The school-based APN was chosen as the person to convey to the CMHC APN information regarding responses to medication and side effects, as well as progress reports. The school team stayed in close contact with the CMHC therapists and met formally every month to discuss Mark's progress. Mark's mother and teachers completed evaluation forms for ADHD; the evaluations indicated strong emotional lability but no attention problems. After Mark's thought processes cleared, he was observed for several months, after which he was determined to have bipolar disorder. His mother, who also had a history of bipolar disorder, was willing to have Mark take a mood stabilizer.

The entire team worked closely and supportively with this family during stable periods as well as during crises. Because of the cooperation and involvement between the school and the CMHC, Mark was able to avoid hospitalization and was maintained in his home. He is learning to read, spell, and do mathematics at his grade level. Although Mark obviously has special needs, of which his classmates are aware, Mark is far more accepted socially. He is no longer delusional and has responded to nonverbal cueing from his teacher when his stories begin to mix fantasy and reality. In addition, Mark's younger sibling has been referred to the Head Start program, and his mother has been referred to the National Alliance for the Mentally Ill for support and education.

To objectively assess the patient's outcome, several areas have been monitored. Mark's school attendance has improved from 79% to 93%. The appropriateness of his responses in classroom activities has improved from 30% to 90%. Mark's overall score on Conners' Rating Scales of hyperactivity and inattention (Conners 1990) has decreased from 82% to 25%. His score on the Global Assessment of Functioning (American Psychiatric Association 2000) improved from 40 to 65.

Theoretical Models

Nurses are frequently involved in the care of children who have been abused physically, sexually, or emotionally or who live in crisis-prone families with multiple problems. In all cases of abuse and in high-risk families, interventions need to focus on prevention of long-term problems. It is important that nurses provide care that is grounded in theory and research, and evaluation must be conducted to demonstrate effective results. Models of particular importance in community settings are the strength-based model and the crisis intervention model. Crisis intervention aims first to stabilize clients so that essential needs are met, then to resolve the crisis and to help them move forward with their life goals. Special skills are needed for working with severely and multiply traumatized clients. Many nurses seek special training for working with victims of rape and sexual abuse. Suicide assessment skills are essential when working in community settings.

The multiple severe crises that many families face can be overwhelming to everyone involved. It is not unusual to work with children and adolescents whose behavior results in frequent suspensions from school and with single-parent families whose members are being stalked and threatened, have experienced physical and sexual abuse, have substance abuse histories, and have mood disorders or anxiety reactions.

In a community setting, it is more helpful to utilize a strength-based model than the traditional problem-focused model. A strength-based model helps instill hope and brings together all of the community resources available for a family. In utilizing a strength-based model, the mental health professional identifies strengths and resources within each functional area (Table 8–3).

TABLE 8–3.   Areas of functioning in a strength-based model

Safety	Spiritual	Academic
Family	Financial	Medical
Social	Judicial	Community

The treatment team then links the family to community resources based on the needs of the individual family. Case managers may be utilized to provide extensive classroom behavior management, to teach effective parenting skills, and to provide assistance to the family in connecting and using available resources. Medication may be helpful in alleviating anxiety and depression and in energizing the parent and child to move forward in attaining goals of therapy. A team approach is illustrated below:

Jerome, 10, and Alisha, 8, were referred to a school-based mental health clinic due to poor school performance, out-of-control behavior, destruction of property, and anxiety symptoms such as hiding under desks and demonstrating an exaggerated startle response. The intake evaluation completed by the clinic social worker revealed that the children lived with their mother and had not had contact with their father in 5 years. The mother was being threatened and followed by her former live-in boyfriend. She reported that her boyfriend used to "hit the kids a lot" when she was at work, which precipitated her asking him to move out after they had lived together for 18 months. The mother also reported that both children frequently have nightmares and wet the bed.

The following family strengths were identified using a strength-based model: the mother is employed and is meeting the family's basic financial needs; the mother has a supportive employer; there is a positive, strong bond between the mother and the children; there is a history of the mother protecting the children and ending an abusive relationship; and the family qualifies for Medicaid, which will reimburse for counseling and medication.

The children were referred to the APN, who diagnosed them with posttraumatic stress disorder and prescribed a selective serotonin reuptake inhibitor for both children. The team met and planned the following multidisciplinary treatment plan:

Social worker: Conduct individual therapy and family therapy; refer mother to abuse survivor group

APN: Prescribe and monitor medications; monitor enuresis

Case manager: Link family to free legal aid and safe after-school program; observe children in classroom; work with mother and teacher on behavior management

Psychologist: Test for learning disabilities

Psychiatrist: Supervise APN and see children every 3 months

Community-Based Team Membership

Community-based nursing often requires the nurse, as well as other professionals, to be members of community-wide crisis intervention teams. This requirement may be particularly difficult because many volunteer lay people are often involved in such teams. These volunteers may have had a role in the development of the team and as a result may feel that they own it to a degree.

Working in any community setting requires an open, nonjudgmental attitude, a high degree of flexibility, tolerance, and excellent communication skills. One must be able to collaborate, solve problems, advocate, and resolve conflicts with other persons and agencies involved with the family or community. Building and maintaining relationships within and between agencies is crucial. Nurses who need or are accustomed to a great deal of control may quickly become frustrated with the need to schedule around court dates, school schedules, and unreliable family transportation or with the obligation to manage or assist in community-wide crises. In such situations, the nurse no longer controls the practice setting but is an invited guest into the community. Without a trusting, respectful relationship, clients and their families will not engage in treatment. Without mutual respect between all community-based personnel, interagency collaboration diminishes and chaos increases in crisis situations; as a result, persons needing treatment may avoid the agency that provides it.

The nurse cannot view himself or herself as the expert on the team but instead must respect the knowledge and expertise of *all* team members. It is important to note that the client may be a family, a school, or the entire community, and all are vital members of the team. When working with families, remember that unless services are court ordered, the parents ultimately make the decision to accept or decline services. In community settings, trusting relationships have a more positive impact than confrontation. To expect absolute compliance is unrealistic and inappropriate. The nursing role on a crisis intervention team is well illustrated by the following example:

> Tina, employed by a community mental health clinic, is also a member of the countywide interdisciplinary mental health crisis intervention team. The team works closely with the Red Cross. The clinic and the Red Cross jointly sponsor disaster training for community volunteers, the police and fire departments, and school personnel. In large-scale disasters, the crisis team works closely with the Red Cross in setting up and maintaining shelters, providing counseling to survivors and disaster victims, and debriefing the crisis workers. The crisis team is activated when crises or emergency situations occur at schools, churches, businesses, or industrial sites and within communities. After an automobile accident in which two high school students were killed, Tina spent most of the day at the students' school. She and two other counselors helped the principal plan and organize an assembly at which all students would be given accurate information about the accident (rumor control), students' questions would be answered, and students would be told where counselors would be in case anyone needed to talk. That day, Tina and her colleagues counseled several students and teachers who had close associations with the boys who had died. They encouraged the distraught teens and teachers to reach out to the families of the deceased teens, to share their feelings of loss, and to help plan the memorial service.

Teenagers and teachers often feel helpless and afraid to interfere in another's grief. Offering them suggestions and helping them make contacts in time of stress helps them build confidence in their ability to be supportive of others and fosters positive community relationships for the youngsters, the school, and the community.

The Prescriptive Authority Role

In response to the growing shortage of child psychiatrists and the increasing availability of safer, more effective medication, many agencies are electing to utilize APNs with authority to prescribe medication for children and adolescents. This occurs especially in community-based settings in underserved rural and inner-city areas. For agencies, hiring an APN rather than a doctor can be a more affordable way to add a staff member who possesses extensive knowledge of medical issues specific to the target population.

To obtain prescriptive authority, APNs must make a separate application to their state licensing board. The application requires documentation of graduate education, continuing education, clinical supervision, and education in psychopharmacology. A collaborative practice agreement with a child psychiatrist is also required. It can take up to 6 months for an APN to obtain his or her first collaborative practice agreement and prescriptive authority certificate. In some states, prescriptive authority is granted along with APN licensure. However, a collaborative relationship with a physician is still required before an APN may prescribe medication. It is wise to submit the applications as quickly as possible to be able to function in the prescriptive role. In the first collaborative agreement, the APN should include a section detailing any training in the prescriptive role that he or she will be receiving from the collaborating physician. Although all APNs receive psychopharmacology training in their graduate program, it is wise from a risk management perspective to obtain additional current training (including consideration of drug interactions) from a child psychiatrist. Presented in Table 8–4 is an example of the information that must be included (requirements vary from state to state) in the written collaborative agreement that enables an APN to have prescriptive authority. It should be noted that APNs may provide therapy independently of a psychiatrist. However, as with all mental health therapy, regular supervision and consultation are recommended and may be required by many agencies and third-party payers.

▎ FINANCIAL REALITIES

Psychiatric nurses practicing in community-based settings must become knowledgeable about and responsible for reimbursement for services. A community-based psychiatric nurse, whether a generalist or an APN, is usually required to bill enough hours to support his or her position. Therefore, nurses must meet specific criteria to be placed on third-party provider panels. For an APN, these criteria usually include appropriate proof of licensure, supervision, a collaborative practice agreement with a child psychiatrist, licensure for prescriptive authority, and often national certification in the subspecialty of child and adolescent psychiatric nursing. Application for provider status with Medicaid and other third-party payers can be a frustrating, lengthy process. It is often helpful to network with other child and adolescent psychiatric APNs in one's geographical area to learn the application and coding practices. In addition, agencies that hire psychiatric APNs should be able to provide resources.

In most states, APNs are authorized by Medicaid to prescribe medication and provide therapy under the supervision of a child psychiatrist. Medicaid also requires that the child psychiatrist regularly evaluate children who are

TABLE 8–4. Content for a written collaborative practice agreement between an advanced practice nurse (APN) and physician

Names of parties to the agreement	Training of the APN in the prescriptive authority role
Titles of parties to the agreement	
Home and business telephone numbers	Collaboration
Home and business addresses	Frequency of physician review of patients
License numbers	
Board certification	Scheduled supervision
All practice locations	Functions to be performed by the APN
Other written practice agreements	
Duration of agreement	Physician's availability for consultation and emergencies, including coverage during vacations and illnesses
Original signatures	

Source. Adapted from Indiana State Board of Nursing: Advanced Practice Nurse Prescriptive Authority. Indianapolis, IN, Indiana Health Professions Bureau, 2005.

taking medication. APNs may provide therapy and prescribe medication for clients who pay out-of-pocket. Clients receiving care from a CMHC are often eligible to be charged fees on a sliding scale based on their income level.

Third-party payers usually require documentation for prior authorization to treat and for continuation of services beyond the authorized number of visits. Nurses who have billing requirements or productivity expectations must adhere to the *Code of Ethics for Nurses* (American Nurses Association 2001) in their billing practices. Patients should receive only the services they need and be billed only for services they receive. Any falsification in documentation or billing is fraudulent and places both the nurse's license and the agency at risk.

Another reality of community-based psychiatric care is the lack of resources available to the treatment team. Mental health nurses who are contracted to work in community settings—such as schools, juvenile centers, or day care settings—often must function in environments that have less than ideal space, privacy, and supplies. A designated telephone line or voice mail system may not be available, nor the luxury of a secretary or a computer. The provision of these items must be clearly delineated when an agency contracts the services of one of its nurses to another setting. It is necessary to specify which resources are needed and available in the contracted practice setting. The nurse must determine the willingness of the agency to provide the resources. Community-based psychiatric nurses must be flexible and considerate in working with agencies to obtain resources in unusual practice settings.

The decision by an agency to provide mental health services to a community-based organization must be carefully determined by the agency's administrators, clinical leaders, and billing specialists. Nurses should be involved in this process and can help their agencies solve problems in finding the needed resources. CMHCs are in a good position to contract for these services because their income from state and local governments can supplement the program initially. Multiple agencies in a community can form partnerships to provide mental health services to underserved areas in their community. Contracts must include details about use of space, technology, personnel, reimbursement, confidentiality, communication with agency staff, and policies regarding management of aggressive behavior by clients—which is especially important given the degree of violence that is being seen in schools today.

▌ REWARDS

Despite limited resources, a community setting can be extremely rewarding to work in. In many ways, the role can be ideal because of the team effort and the possibility for communication with other significant people in the child's life, such as teachers. Child and adolescent psychiatric nurses can provide valuable information to other disciplines about how to interact more effectively with these often challenging children. Psychiatric nurses in these settings can learn from professionals in other disciplines and can gain a clearer understanding of the multiple issues that affect clients. Psychiatric nurses can have a broader impact by consulting with and educating other professionals about the mental health needs of children. Great satisfaction can be found in helping children improve their daily functioning and increase their options in life and in helping families be more effective and less dysfunctional. In addition, the nurse in this setting can provide excellent, affordable care to extremely ill clients who would otherwise not receive any services.

▌ CHALLENGES

Additional specific challenges are inherent to working in community-based outpatient settings. These include safety issues, confidentiality, appropriate releases for communication, observation of nontherapeutic behavior by others working with one's clients, and when and how to refer patients to more restrictive environments when they are no longer appropriate for an outpatient program. Each setting, job, and role brings its own particular set of challenges.

Safety should be the overriding priority of every agency and of each professional. Policies should be in place for assessing, preventing, and de-escalating aggression and for dealing with a multitude of unsafe situations. Staff members should receive regular training on the prevention and management of aggression. Staff members should not be expected to go into unknown, potentially unsafe environments. For example, scheduling a first meeting with a client in the client's home is inadvisable. The professional should first meet with the client in a safe setting and assess the home environment in terms of safety. During an intake evaluation, the nurse should conduct a safety assessment in terms of both visiting the client at home and meeting alone with the client in the agency. The most common predictor of violent behavior is a history of such behavior. The community-based psychiatric nurse should assess all persons living in the home for past violence. The nurse should also assess for the presence of weapons, for the use of drugs and alcohol, the number of people who live in and visit the home, the probability that illicit drug sales are taking place, and the general condition of the neighborhood.

A nurse should never conduct a meeting in a client's home if he or she feels unsafe there. If the nurse does not have an office in which to meet clients, meetings can be scheduled at a local library or restaurant. If, at any time during a home visit, drug or alcohol use occurs, the visit should be terminated due to the unpredictability of behavior resulting from such substance use. The agency should also provide its staff with cellular phones to further address the safety of its personnel. Of course, many neighborhoods are unsafe after dark. In addition, the nurse must use safety precautions when going from the agency to the parking area. It is not advisable to stay after dark to finish charting or to meet with clients, either at the agency or in the client's home.

Client confidentiality can also be complicated. Confidentiality must always be maintained, but gray areas exist once releases of information have been signed. For example, a signed release for the nurse to share information with agency personnel does not permit the nurse to share that information with persons who are not involved in the care of the client. It is also unwise to give detailed psychiatric histories or information about the client's diagnosis or past abuse, particularly if the agency personnel must interact with the alleged perpetrator. Even with a signed release, any information that is shared should be general and should be focused on how that professional can better interact with the client. If the nurse feels strongly that a team member who is not a mental health professional needs more detailed information, the nurse can schedule a meeting between all parties involved and let the legal guardian share the information. Remember that not all professionals have the same expectation and training in terms of confidentiality and boundaries.

One of the most difficult situations to handle is the witnessing of nontherapeutic or even emotionally abusive treatment of children in the setting in which the nurse works. A community-based nurse will often be working under contract in an agency and may be the only mental health professional (or one of few) in that location. How then does the nurse address the negative behavior while still maintaining strong enough relationships within the agency to be effective in that role? Above all, the nurse must be a client advocate. However, the nurse cannot change the behavior of all other workers in the setting. Each person varies in his or her willingness to accept feedback. At times, the best the nurse can do is to provide a role model of more appropriate behavior, provide in-service consultations on behavior management or other topics, or work closely with the manager of the agency. Physical abuse, however, must be reported to appropriate authorities. Dealing with these situations requires a great deal of tact, maturity, and excellent communication skills.

Finally, knowing when to refer a client to more restrictive and intensive treatment is often difficult. The community agency may be unwilling to do so either because of financial responsibilities or because of differing values or goals (e.g., to maintain family unity). However, if the client cannot be safely maintained in an outpatient setting, the team has an ethical responsibility to attempt to refer the client to protect the safety of others. Often the client can be maintained in the home but can be referred to a more restrictive school or day treatment program. At other times, the client may need an even more restrictive environment. The situation can become very complicated because of factors such as program availability, payment sources, and transportation. In addition, the client and family may refuse the team's recommendation. If such refusal occurs, the team must very clearly document its recommendations for the client and the family's choice. Discussing the case with the agency's risk management team is also wise. In some severe instances, when families refuse to acknowledge the danger and do not follow recommendations for treatment or referrals, the most therapeutic course of action is to terminate services to that client. In such an event, the client and family must be given a list of more appropriate treatment options so that the client is not being abandoned.

▌ CONCLUSIONS

The standard for delivery of psychiatric care to children and adolescents has changed dramatically from inpatient hospitalization to a more community-based model. Child and adolescent psychiatric nurses have many new and exciting roles available in this practice setting. Nurses bring a wealth of knowledge to the treatment team and to their clients. APNs in particular are being sought out to fill a need in underserved inner-city and rural settings. Under the supervision of a physician, APNs can provide affordable, highly skilled medication management and therapy. Working in a community setting offers a unique set of rewards and challenges. Because resources are often limited, nurses must be clinically competent, exercise good judgment, and be very flexible. Nurses must be able to establish and maintain good relationships with team members in their own settings and with other involved agencies. With the recent national focus on the emotional needs of youths, opportunities exist for creative, highly skilled nurses to have a strong, positive impact in communities.

▌ REFERENCES

American Nurses Association: Code of Ethics for Nurses, With Interpretive Statements. Washington, DC, American Nurses Publishing, 2001

American Psychiatric Association: Diagnostic and Statistical Manual of Mental Disorders, 4th Edition, Text Revision. Washington, DC, American Psychiatric Association, 2000

Conners KC: Manual for Connors' Rating Scales: Conners' Teacher Rating Scale, Conners' Parent Rating Sale. North Tonawanda, NY, Multi-Health Systems, Inc., 1990

Worley NK (ed): Mental Health Nursing in the Community. St Louis, MO, CV Mosby, 1997

▌ SUGGESTED READINGS

Austin JK: Behavior problems in children with epilepsy, in Psychiatric–Mental Health Nursing: Integrating the Behavioral and Biological Sciences. Edited by McBride AB, Austin JK. Philadelphia, PA, WB Saunders, 1996, pp 107–132

Billings CV: Psychiatric–mental health nursing: 2000 and beyond, in Comprehensive Psychiatric Nursing, 5th Edition. Edited by Haber J, Krainovich-Miller B, Leach-McMahon A, et al. St. Louis, MO, CV Mosby, 1997, pp 16–29

Burgess AW, Hartmann CR: Rape trauma and posttraumatic stress disorder, in Psychiatric–Mental Health Nursing: Integrating the Behavioral and Biological Sciences. Edited by McBride AB, Austin JK. Philadelphia, PA, WB Saunders, 1996, pp 53–81

Burgess AW, Hartmann CR, Clements PT: Treating child sexual trauma, in Psychiatric Nursing: Promoting Mental Health. Edited by Burgess BW. Stamford, CT, Appleton & Lange, 1996, pp 53–81

Caplan G: Principles of Preventive Psychiatry. New York, Basic Books, 1964

Fagin CM (ed): Foreword, in Readings in Child and Adolescent Psychiatric Nursing. St. Louis, MO, CV Mosby, 1974, pp 1–5

Hardin SB: Catastrophic stress, in Psychiatric–Mental Health Nursing: Integrating the Behavioral and Biological Sciences. Edited by McBride AB, Austin JK. Philadelphia, PA, WB Saunders, 1996, pp 82–106

Johnson BS: Mental health of children, adolescents, and families, in Child, Adolescent, and Family Psychiatric Nursing. Edited by Johnson BS. Philadelphia, PA, JB Lippincott, 1995, pp 3–14

McBride AB: Psychiatric–mental health nursing in the twenty-first century, in Psychiatric–Mental Health Nursing: Integrating the Behavioral and Biological Sciences. Edited by McBride AB, Austin JK. Philadelphia, PA, WB Saunders, 1996, pp 1–10

McBride AB, Austin JK: Integrating the behavioral and biological sciences: implications for practice, education, and research, in Psychiatric–Mental Health Nursing: Integrating the Behavioral and Biological Sciences. Edited by McBride AB, Austin JK. Philadelphia, PA, WB Saunders, 1996, pp 425–434

Stanley SR: Trends in mental health care of children, adolescents, and families, in Child, Adolescent, and Family Psychiatric Nursing. Edited by Johnson BS. Philadelphia, PA, JB Lippincott, 1996

West P, Evans CL: The specialty of child and adolescent psychiatric nursing, in Psychiatric and Mental Health Nursing With Children and Adolescents. Edited by West P, Evans CLS. Gaithersburg, MD, Aspen, 1992

Worley NK, Owens VJ: Schools, in Mental Health Nursing in the Community. Edited by Worley NK. St Louis, MO, CV Mosby, 1997, pp 226–238

PART
III

Interdisciplinary Functioning in
the Community Setting

9 COMMUNITY MENTAL HEALTH CENTERS

Carlos Salguero, M.D., M.P.H., F.A.P.A.

The present-day community mental health center (CMHC) and related agencies are diversified and provide comprehensive mental health services for children. Their methods of delivering services to children and their families have changed drastically since the 1980s because of the interplay of a number of factors discussed in this chapter. The modern CMHC–considered to be part of a continuum of care–represents a dynamic, highly specialized entity in which consultants and staff work together to provide broad services to children and their families. In this chapter, the administrative and clinical structure and functions of a CMHC are described, in addition to ways in which professionals might envision their role in a CMHC and its system.

In association with other community agencies, the CMHC plays a pivotal role in a continuum-of-care model. The Village for Families and Children in Hartford, Connecticut, is an example. With 350 employees and an annual budget of more than $10 million, it provides an array of services to more than 2,550 children a year. Its facilities and services include a safe home for children who are under state custody, a subacute inpatient unit, a 10-bed diagnostic unit, intensive family services, foster care, extended day treatment, outpatient education and treatment, school-based clinics, services to children affected by human immunodeficiency virus (HIV) and acquired immunodeficiency syndrome (AIDS), wraparound services, and family resource centers. The services are provided in different sectors of the city to allow easier access by families.

As another example, the Child and Family Guidance Clinic at Hill Health Center, a federally qualified health center in one of the poorest neighborhoods of New Haven, Connecticut, is part of the Behavioral Health Division of the center. The clinic acts as an umbrella for the mental health services of three programs: four school-based clinics, an early intervention program for more than 100 children who are eligible for the Birth to Three program, and the child psychiatry clinic proper. The Birth to Three program is federally funded through the Individuals With Disabilities Education Act; it provides comprehensive services for children from birth to 36 months of age who exhibit moderate to significant developmental delays due to specific medical and cognitive impairments. The child psychiatry clinic interfaces with other Hill Health Center services—for example, providing consultation-liaison with the pediatrics department; the Special Supplemental Nutrition Program for Women, Infants, and Children; and the perinatal unit attached to the obstetrics and gynecology department. Contrasting organizational charts for these agencies are presented in Figures 9–1 and 9–2.

The two community clinics described represent comprehensive, coordinated, multiagency therapeutic approaches to deal with the mental health problems faced by children as part of a continuum-of-care network in their respective catchment areas.

▌ THE CHILD SECTION OF A CMHC

The child section of a CMHC provides services to a catchment area as defined by its licensing source, often a specific state agency such as the department of mental health (in Connecticut, it is the Department of Children and Families). In addition to CMHCs, the state may issue licensure or approval for freestanding child guidance clinics and child psychiatry clinics at medical schools, hospitals, or other facilities licensed to provide psychiatric services for children. The budget that supports the clinic activities may be derived from the clinic's licensing source; from patient fees; and from private, local, state, or federal grants that allow the clinic to provide a broad array of mental health services. Patient fees may come from family self-payment, third-party private insurance, or managed care organizations (MCOs). Contracts with MCOs are often for the provision of services to families on Medicaid, to indigent recipients who are covered under some entitlement program, or to participants in special programs. Charitable agencies (e.g., the United Way) add to the agency budget and allow CMHCs to use a sliding scale for children whose parents are not covered by insurance or by Medicaid managed care. The consultant or CMHC staff should have a basic understanding of the role of managed care in the provision of mental health services to families.

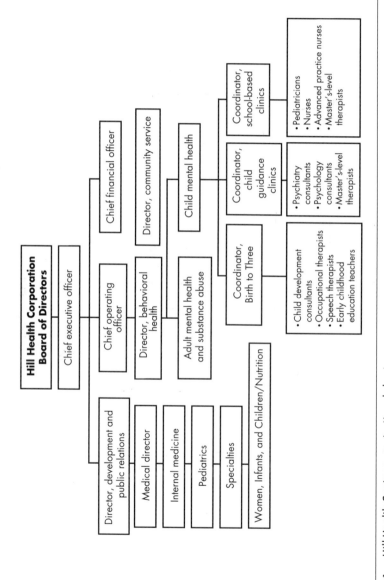

FIGURE 9–1. Hill Health Center organizational chart.

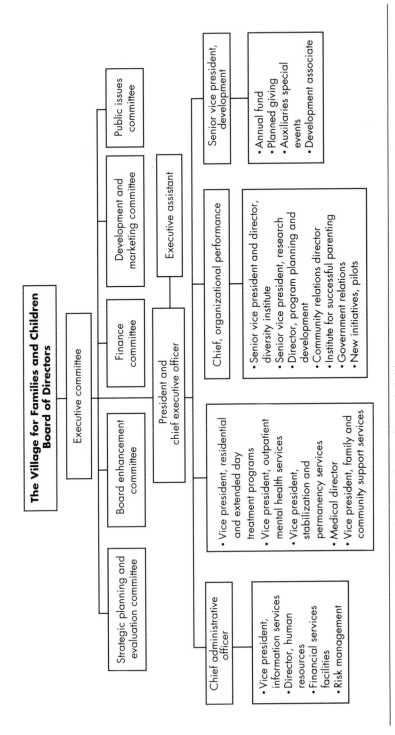

FIGURE 9–2. Organizational chart for the Village for Families and Children.

▌ CMHC GOVERNANCE AND ROLE STRUCTURE

Different configurations exist for CMHC governance (e.g., whom the director reports to). For most CMHCs and freestanding, nonprofit mental health clinics, a *governing* board of directors hires the clinic director. The board is responsible for the overall solvency of the clinic and for ensuring that the mission of the clinic is maintained. A CMHC *advisory* board of directors does not have such decision-making power. Instead, the power to make such decisions is vested elsewhere (e.g., county commissioners or boards, university or medical school boards, or the commissioner of mental health).

The staff of a CMHC or a child clinic may be unionized. The union enters into contract negotiations every 1, 2, or 3 years with the board and the administration. Negotiations involve salaries, fringe benefits, staff hiring, and the like. When applying for employment, prospective professional staff members or consultants should be aware of the latest agency audit or should request a copy. They should become acquainted with the organizational structure of the agency, including the makeup of the board and whether any issues or concerns seem to stand out.

Staffing at a CMHC

The configuration of a CMHC child section depends on its size and the comprehensiveness of its services. The child section is generally staffed in the following manner: a director or chief of children's services; an associate director for clinical services or a clinical director; program directors; supervisory staff, who are usually licensed master's- or doctorate-level professionals; and front-line staff, who may be baccalaureate- or master's-level social workers, psychologists, marriage and family therapists, and nurses. In some CMHCs, a position of medical director exists, especially when it is required by state regulation. The descriptive functions of the director, clinical director, child mental health professionals, and child psychiatrist follow.

Director

The director of children's services, who holds the most critical position in the clinic, is usually a social worker or psychologist with many years of experience in administrative leadership. A child psychiatrist or nurse may serve as director, but this seldom happens. Many clinics cannot afford to pay a sufficient salary to have a child psychiatrist as their full-time director. Exceptions exist, especially if the clinic is part of an academic institution, in which case a faculty child psychiatrist may assume this function. In broad terms, the director is responsible for the smooth operation of the clinic in its provision of services to children and families, whether these are direct clinical or specialized services; the director also oversees the hiring of staff who will provide clinical services and administrative support. Clinically, the most important task for the director is to establish quality and productivity standards for the staff, following the licensing and quality assurance standards established by the agency. Productivity standards are closely linked to the clinic's operating budget. Critical functions for the director are actively representing the clinic at state and community levels and, in concert with other related agencies, initiating and coordinating a better system of care for the catchment area.

Given their background and experience, CMHC child section directors may be key persons in the hierarchy of the agency or may simply follow major decisions made by the CMHC director. Although an important component of the CMHC, the child clinic may be the most vulnerable component when budgetary decisions are made. The director of the child section reports to the CMHC director, who in turn may report to the funding and licensing state agency or to a board of directors.

The director of children's services, whose leadership sets the tone for the overall function of the clinic, should be resourceful, creative, well trained in clinical and administrative matters, and attuned to the needs of the clinic. He or she must understand the many facets of managed care and the politics of mental health at the state and local levels. Because of the complex operation of many services under many programs, often for a very diverse population, the director also needs to have a keen understanding of the community and the clientele served by the clinic. Like an orchestra conductor who knowledgably and passionately unifies different musicians who contribute to an effective and moving work of music, the director of children's services must know how to manage and guide his or her staff to provide quality services.

Clinical Director

The director of children's services delegates clinical responsibilities to the clinical director, who is usually a licensed psychologist or licensed social worker. Because the clinical director runs the everyday affairs of the clinic, this position requires significant administrative and clinical experience. The clinical director ensures that the provision of clinical services to children and their families follows professional, ethical, and legal standards or guidelines. These standards or guidelines are usually stipulated by the state's department of mental health or the agency that licenses the clinic. The clinical director should supervise every aspect of the process of evaluating, diagnosing, and treating children and their families. The clinical director chairs the clinical team or teams that periodically review all new and ongoing cases or delegates this function to a senior clinician. In university-based clinics, a child psychiatrist or other professional (psychologist or social worker) with experience on the clinical faculty may chair the team. The clinical director establishes the standards for treatment to be performed at the clinic and the guidelines for clinical supervision of every clinician who performs clinical services. Some of the functions of the director of child services (e.g., hiring staff, implementing productivity standards, and ensuring the smooth functioning of the clinic) can be delegated to the clinical director. The clinical director may coordinate a number of programs and hire program directors to manage these programs. The director and the clinical director must have a good working relationship. Their views on staff development and training, philosophy, and quality of treatment should be complementary to ensure that the clinic staff feel motivated to work and professionally fulfilled.

Child Mental Health Professionals

Each child clinic has its own unique staffing configuration designed to run the clinical programs for the population that it serves. The job description for each clinical staff or consultant position should detail the responsibilities of the position and the required training, experience, and professional credentials. At the Village for Families and Children, the director of all children's services and programs is a master's-level licensed psychiatric social worker. Children's programs and the child psychiatry section report to her. The director reports to the chief operating officer. Most of the professionals providing outpatient services are social workers and marriage and family therapists, whereas in subacute units (a step down from hospital services), nurses, psychologists, child psychiatrists, and social workers form the core of the treatment team. It is essential that clinic professionals be well trained for the services they are to provide. They need to know the standards of practice for the clinic, who established the standards, and whether the clinic's standards are compatible with ethical standards and treatment parameters established by their own professional associations. The director of children's services must make the fundamental decisions concerning which professionals to hire and which discipline or person can function most effectively within the constraints of the budget assigned to the clinic. For example, baccalaureate-level case managers can perform adequately in some instances; they can even provide outstanding performance following up on patients in the community compared with social workers with master's degrees. The job description for a case manager may specify that only a bachelor's degree is required. Some parent aide programs only require staff members to have an associate's degree. Some clinics use advanced practice nurses to prescribe psychotropic medication under the supervision of a child and adolescent psychiatrist.

Child Psychiatrist

The following services are provided by both staff and consulting child psychiatrists:

- Perform psychiatric evaluations of children.
- Evaluate the need for medication in children and then prescribe it and monitor it.
- Sign off on treatment plans if required.
- Participate in committees in which the presence of the child psychiatrist is needed.
- Provide or participate in supervision of clinical staff.
- Coordinate and supervise the training and supervision of child and general psychiatry residents or other trainees placed at the clinic, as appropriate.
- Provide consultation to the different programs functioning under the umbrella of the CMHC.

Child psychiatrists who are members of the CMHC staff have different roles than those who are consultants. Some of the differences relate to the number of hours worked at the clinic. As employees of the CMHC, staff psychiatrists are an integral part of the clinic and are influential members of the clinic's hierarchy. Their responsibilities are dictated by and go beyond other needs of the clinic than the responsibilities of a consulting child psychiatrist. The performance of the consulting child psychiatrist is clearly delineated in his or her contract with the agency. He or she is being asked to provide expertise in a special area of consultation. The consulting child psychiatrist has the opportunity to perform in multiple roles as delineated in Chapter 5, "Role of the Child and Adolescent Psychiatrist."

Service Delivery Models

The clinician working as a consultant or a staff member at a CMHC may be providing services at several levels of care (from outpatient care, emergency mobile psychiatric services, and extended day treatment to respite care and family preservation programs). Yet to be more effective in their role, clinicians and administrators must keep the following in mind: 1) the psychosocial makeup of the population in the catchment area (e.g., whether the population is predominantly middle class, on welfare, rural, urban, Asian, Hispanic, and so forth); and 2) the predominant issues facing the community, especially regarding children.

In the model of a clinic located in the inner city, the director and administrative leadership must be cognizant of the problems faced by the catchment area population, such as high unemployment and high prevalence of parents with substance abuse problems. Likewise, many parents have very low self-esteem and face excessive stress in their everyday lives. They feel as if they are being scrutinized by the state worker or similar person of authority, by the protective services worker, by the teacher, and even by personnel from the primary care clinic they attend. In such clinics, gang membership, teenage pregnancy, homicide, juvenile delinquency, and school suspensions occur more often than in other sectors of the community. The CMHC must use a model to best meet the needs of the population it serves. The clinic administration or consultant must consider similar issues for isolated rural areas and be mindful of the everyday realities faced by some families in the community. These include being late for appointments because transportation is unavailable and being unable to come for appointments because there is no babysitter to care for their other children. Sometimes the parents do not have a telephone to call the clinic to cancel and reschedule an appointment. Some clinics hire an outreach worker or case manager to visit the family at home and remind family members of their appointments, check compliance with medication regimens, and arrange for transportation services. Given the crisis orientation of many referred families, new patients should ideally be screened immediately, within a week for urgent referrals, to ascertain if immediate help is needed.

An important strategy to reduce the budget-busting no-show/cancellation rate is to develop a flexible schedule of appointments and a walk-in clinic for unscheduled patients, patients who are known not to come to their regularly scheduled appointments, patients seeking services for the first time, and emergencies. The walk-in clinic can function as a screening tool and can be used for immediate intervention with families who need only one session to deal with a problem for which they want advice or advocacy (e.g., making a call to the state worker, principal, or teacher or referring the family to another appropriate facility for follow-up). This model is illustrated below:

> A parent came to the walk-in clinic for the first time to seek assistance in dealing with her 7-year-old son's school. She felt that her son had been unfairly suspended for 3 days for running out of the school grounds. As the evaluator on call listened to the mother's story, it became clear to him that the son was an impulsive child who needed a full evaluation. The evaluator called the school social worker to discuss the case, and the child was able to return to school the next day. Soon afterward, the clinician called the principal and explained the nature of the child's behavior. The principal was satisfied with the clinician's explanation. Plans for evaluation and treatment were made by the treatment team that same week.

In a second model, a clinic providing services to middle-class or working-class children may offer a different set of services than one in the inner city.

For this clientele, transportation to the clinic is not a problem. Families mostly come on time and like to be seen on time. The problems faced by clinics serving middle-class or working-class children may be due to different factors than those seen in the inner-city clinic, but they nevertheless deserve as much attention. Parental divorce, custody, domestic violence, family conflicts, and substance abuse are clinical entities seen at clinics that cater to a more working-class or middle-class community, and these issues are addressed with relevant programs.

In a third model, professionals working with Native American children should know that these children appear to be at higher risk than other racial or ethnic groups in the United States for mental health problems, including depression, substance abuse, suicide, and homicide. These children grow up in communities with high rates of unemployment, poverty, outdated and often irrelevant educational systems, and stressful home lives plagued by broken nuclear and extended family networks. Therefore, broad-based preventive measures and public health promotion approaches by a clinic will be the most effective, cost-efficient means to reduce the incidence and prevalence of mental health problems in the shortest period of time (Barlow and Walkup 1998; see also Chapter 2, "Public-Sector Dynamics for Child Mental Health"). Issues concerning the rural model of service delivery are described more fully elsewhere (Barlow and Walkup 1998; see also Chapter 4, "Practical Aspects of Rural Mental Health Care").

These examples of service delivery models highlight the different needs of populations in different geographical catchment areas and the necessity of clinics to be attuned to the needs and situations of their clientele. The cultural context in which services are planned and implemented is also critical. In the inner city, the walk-in clinic responds to the crisis orientation that many families exhibit. In a rural area, providing mental health services in the schools can be more effective; it enables meeting the child in an environment where he or she feels comfortable and engaging the family in a preferable and less stigmatizing location than the CMHC.

Table 9–1 highlights some of the characteristics exhibited and issues faced by four types of mental health care systems for children and adolescents: urban inner-city clinics and services, urban-suburban clinics and services, rural mental health services, and Native American services. Ideally, all should strive to implement a fully integrated continuum of care in which treatment proceeds from the most restrictive, expensive intensive care (such as that provided by psychiatric hospitals and residential treatment centers) to a moderately intense mode (such as family preservation services, respite care, and subacute care) to the least intense mode, in which community-based programs (such as those provided by CMHCs and freestanding child guidance clinics and school-based clinics) provide services that are integrated with linkages between child-caring agencies and programs and mechanisms for planning, developing, and coordinating services.

▌ NEEDS ASSESSMENT

The foundation of a needs assessment is composed of 1) the process of answering the questions concerning the socioeconomic and ethnic makeup of the population seen at the clinic (posed above under "Service Delivery Models"), and 2) the strengths and resources represented in that population. An effective assessment provides direction for developing or modifying policies and procedures and for seeking the required financial resources to fund new programs or new procedures. Local foundations or charitable organizations such as the United Way may be the logical sources to turn to, whereas in other instances the clinic may have to advocate with the state to obtain the necessary funding to carry out the services needed.

Equally critical to conducting a needs assessment is tracking the outcomes of planned changes that result from CMHC staff work with clients. The objectives and outcomes of service must be detailed. In the inner city, a decrease in the no-show rate might result in fewer children dropping out of school and better consumer satisfaction. In a rural community, an increase in the number of children seen may indicate greater accessibility to services.

The director and staff of the CMHC must bring agency developments before the public and policy makers. The CMHC director or staff can write a column for the local newspaper to promote an activity, appear on local radio and television, and host open houses of the CMHC to accomplish this objective. The CMHC director and staff can also approach foundations and local charities that are interested in a particular mental health issue. Centers can forge alliances with other community agencies and advocacy groups. Parents can also actively request changes in state mental health policy for children so that more children can be seen and helped.

Moreover, as greater numbers of minority groups obtain access to mental health services, CMHCs must become more sensitive to the social and cultural issues of the population being served. Families come with their own beliefs about mental illness and their own expectations for treatment. To better treat these populations, it is important for a clinic to become culturally competent. This competence can be accomplished by administrators and clinicians attending to the influence of cultural patterns on family health-seeking behavior and how sociocultural context can affect symptoms. In Latino adolescents, for example, somatic anxiety is better accepted by families than other symptoms of distress. Culturally competent staff members, from the receptionist to chief executive officer, must understand and utilize this dynamic

TABLE 9–1. Child mental health service delivery models for different populations

Characteristics and issues	Service delivery model			
	Urban inner-city clinic	Urban-suburban clinic	Rural	Native American
Population composition	Mostly African American, Hispanic minorities	White and some minorities	White and some new immigrant groups	Native American
Socioeconomic status	Poor; many below poverty level and receiving some type of federal or state assistance	Working class Unemployed Some Medicaid recipients	Poor; some partial employment, low income levels	Poor
Most prevalent community mental health issues	High unemployment Substance abuse Gangs, teenage pregnancy, urban violence, juvenile delinquency, and high drop out rate from middle school and high school	Parental divorce Family custody conflicts Unemployment Domestic violence Substance and alcohol abuse	Limited tolerance of diversity and deviance Fear, misunderstanding, and stigmatization of mental illness Isolated communities	Alcoholism Substance abuse Higher rates of unemployment Suicide, homicide Stressful home lives
Treatment options	Several using continuum-of-care model	Several using continuum-of-care model	Few Fragmented continuum of care; increased responsibility for schools and pediatricians	Very few No continuum of care

TABLE 9–1. Child mental health service delivery models for different populations *(continued)*

Characteristics and issues	Service delivery model			
	Urban inner-city clinic	Urban-suburban clinic	Rural	Native American
Therapies mostly used	Western-based models Crisis intervention Psychotherapy outreach Medication management	Western-based models Psychotherapy Crisis intervention Medication management	Traditional face-to-face visits not used as often Telemedicine: delivery by telephone and e-mail	Relational worldviews Balance or harmony of multiple interrelating variables Indigenous remedies
Child psychiatrists participating in services	Acceptable number Budget constraints limit participation	Acceptable number Budget constraints limit participation	Few	Almost none
Ancillary supports to treatment	Widely used State and federally funded programs Schools, early intervention programs, and social and youth service agencies	Widely used State and federally funded programs Schools, early intervention programs, and social and youth service agencies	Schools Churches Community organizations	Healers Family members

TABLE 9–1. Child mental health service delivery models for different populations *(continued)*

	Service delivery model			
Characteristics and issues	Urban inner-city clinic	Urban-suburban clinic	Rural	Native American
Barriers to access to mental health services	Poverty Lack of transportation Crowded housing Lack of minority professionals Long waiting lists for services	Lack of health insurance Cost containment by managed care organizations Long waiting lists for services	Lack of transportation to treatment facilities Lack of health insurance Long distances to care facilities	Poverty No fully integrated continuum of care Not enough Native American mental health professionals Reservation health clinics understaffed
Recommended improvements	Increase funding to state agencies to improve continuum of care, especially in prevention programs, school-based clinics, and walk-in clinics and social programs Reduce number of suspensions by schools	Increase funding to state agencies to improve continuum of care Optimize communication between health, mental health, and juvenile justice agencies to assist high-risk youths	Develop better continuum-of-care system using local community agencies and staff from schools, day care centers, and hospitals Provide more incentives for professionals to work in rural areas Increase number of school-based clinics	Develop integrated culturally bound continuum of care Significantly increase funding for preventive public health and mental health programs Increase number of school-based clinics and recreational outlets

to help the youths and their families. Likewise, understanding the cultural conflict experienced by Native American youngsters is critical for their care. Moreover, a reasonable matching of patients with clinicians of the same or similar culture or clinicians skillful in cross-cultural diagnosis and treatment would be prudent.

■ CLINICAL ACTIVITIES AT THE CMHC

Having reviewed the basic setup of the CMHC, its staffing, and the role of managed care, the consultant or staff member working at a CMHC can now better grasp the existing clinical activities that guide the child and the family who enter the CMHC system. Clinicians should review the descriptions of CMHC activities in this section and compare them with the activities of the clinic where they work or plan to work. The intake process is critical to clinic functions, because it often represents the first contact by the person requesting services. Whether the person calls or comes to the clinic in person, a staff member's sensitive, empathic response to an inquiry can allay any initial bias, guilt, or anxiety the person may have. The clinician must elicit the presenting problem or chief complaint before he or she can decide when and how to take action. The child and the family should be given an orientation to the clinic and its procedures. This orientation can be accomplished by placing videotapes and information sheets (e.g., Facts for Families) in the waiting room.

Each CMHC program has its own delivery model. For example, in an outpatient clinic, the evaluation process is most often conducted by a master's-level clinician using a standardized format for that clinic. The format should meet standards set by state and professional accrediting bodies (e.g., the Joint Commission on Accreditation of Healthcare Organizations; JCAHO), regardless of the CMHC's orientation. Each center has its own system of assigning cases. In some centers, a team of master's-level clinicians, licensed psychologists, and child psychiatrists performs an evaluation. The case is then transferred to a therapist. In other clinics, the case is assigned to the therapist from the very beginning. The therapist then makes referrals to other professionals as he or she sees fit.

Case review and follow-up are usually performed in outpatient clinics on a weekly basis. The case management team, under the direction of the clinical director or team leader, provides the guidelines for evaluation and intervention. Measurement of treatment effectiveness is assuming increasing importance. JCAHO is demanding that outcome measures be included in the structure and process of care.

∎ PROGRAM REVIEW

Perhaps the most important questions raised by consultants or professional staff should concern how and to what extent the CMHC meets the goals detailed in its mission statement. How does the agency monitor and use data concerning staff and client satisfaction, staff productivity, and staff development? Does the clinic have a waiting list, and if so, why? Is the population facing barriers to treatment, and if so, what are the strategies to overcome these barriers? Are programs meeting their goals? Is the clinic on a firm footing financially? How is the CMHC functioning in relation to the community? In summary, the clinician must be aware of the CMHC's current functioning and how the CMHC will project itself into the future.

∎ CONCLUSIONS

- The CMHC is an essential part of a coordinated system of care and can provide a wide spectrum of services along a continuum-of-care model.
- Professionals who are considering employment on staff or as consultants at a CMHC need to be acquainted with the new mental health care initiatives, the coordinated systems of care, the economics that affect the system, and the different programs and activities at the CMHC.
- Public-sector psychiatry is a challenging adventure.
- Professionals must deal with barriers to the provision of services and pressures to see more patients in less time; they must also become advocates or educate legislators.
- The new mental health system of care is a step in the right direction because more children are entering the system regardless of race and regardless of social, cultural, and economic background.

∎ REFERENCE

Barlow A, Walkup J: Developing mental health services for Native American children. Child Adolesc Psychiatr Clin N Am 7:555–577, 1998

∎ SUGGESTED READINGS

Bickman L, Heflinger C, Pion G, et al: Evaluation planning for an innovative children's mental health system. Clin Psychol Rev 12:853–865, 1992

Esser G, Schmidt MH, Woerner W: Epidemiology and causes of psychiatric disorders in school-age children: results of a longitudinal study. J Child Psychol Psychiatry 31:243–263, 1990

Kashani JH, Orvaschel H, Rosenberg T, et al: Psychopathology in a community sample of children and adolescents: a developmental perspective. J Am Acad Child Adolesc Psychiatry 28:701–706, 1989

Knitzer J: Unclaimed Children: The Failure of Public Responsibility to Children and Adolescents in Need of Mental Health Services. Washington, DC, Children's Defense Fund, 1982

Stroul BA, Friedman RM: A System of Care for Children and Youth With Severe Emotional Disturbances. Washington, DC, Georgetown University Child Development Center, CASSP Technical Assistance Center, 1986

10 SCHOOLS

Lance D. Clawson, M.D., F.A.A.C.A.P.

The practice of mental health consultation to schools has come of age. School consultation is a form of mental health/human services consultation that originally grew out of the pioneering work of Caplan and coworkers (Caplan and Caplan 1993), who devised ways to work with the huge population of Jewish war orphans after World War II. Psychiatrist Irving N. Berlin (1974) later built on Caplan's principles of consultation, systematically applying them to school settings. Psychiatrists, social workers, psychiatric nurses, and psychologists are increasingly involved in providing mental health consultation to schools as the need for psychological expertise and services within the educational system is becoming widely publicized. This chapter presents an introduction to the tools, knowledge, and attitudes that the individual school consultant must have readily available. An appendix of glossary terms is included at the end of this chapter for quick reference.

∎ THE SCHOOL SETTING

Child and adolescent mental health professionals need a basic understanding of the general structure of their local school system, the roles of various school personnel, the public laws mandating that all children receive an appropriate education, and the "personality" or culture of the school or schools where they will work.

School Personality

Each school and school system has its own approach and attitude toward identification and management of emotionally disturbed youths. This "school personality" frequently reflects the willingness or resistance of the staff to include outside consultants in their inner workings and their ability to identify emotional problems in their pupils. Individuals in leadership positions (e.g., principals and superintendents) often shape this personality. Their interest in emotionally disturbed children and their desire to embrace this population have a broad influence on how a particular school or entire school system provides for special education students. Many pressures on schools exist and may vary by state and locale. Challenges for schools include budget cuts and pressures to raise local scores on standardized tests or to reduce class size. These issues all have impacts on the time, attention, and resources available to address special education needs. School mental health consultants must be aware of these larger systemic and cultural issues as well as school-specific problems to be able to realistically set short- and long-term goals for their consultation.

Public Law

In 1954, the U.S. Supreme Court established the principle of "equal educational opportunity" for all students regardless of any disability. The Education of the Handicapped Act of 1965 (P.L. 89-313) and its 1966 amendments (P.L. 89-750; Title VI) provided for funds to assist states in developing and expanding programs for the education of handicapped students ages 3–21 years. The Education for All Handicapped Children Act of 1975 (P.L. 94-142) required all states to adopt policies and methods to ensure that a free and "appropriate" public education was available to all students. This law mandated that each student in need of special education services be given an Individual Educational Plan (IEP), that the family be involved throughout the process, and that due process rights were guaranteed if the family should disagree with the outcome.

More recent changes include the amendments of 1986 (P.L. 99-457), which established a state grant program for the purpose of providing early intervention services to disabled children from birth to 2 years. The 1990 amendments, the Individuals With Disabilities Education Act (P.L. 101-476), emphasizes meeting the needs of minorities with disabilities, improving personnel recruitment and retention, providing transition services, and advancing early intervention services (Arnold et al. 1993).

Roles and Skills of School Personnel

The consultant must have a good understanding of the different skills and abilities of various school staff members. The consultant must tailor recommendations so that they take into account the role and skills of the consultee and so that they are developmentally appropriate for the children and the school in question (e.g., the developmental progression of children creates shifting expectations for teachers, counselors, and other school staff members across age groups, because teachers have less time available to give to any one student as the students progress to middle and high school). Teachers are the front line of the educational system. They have the greatest exposure to the largest number of students and generally have the best overall knowledge about the students whom they teach. In the course of consultation, information provided by the teacher about a particular student is often invaluable. Although their psychological training is usually limited, teachers usually observe a great deal about their students. A teacher's ability and motivation to carry out a consultant's recommendations (if properly operationalized) is often the make-or-break keystone for any plan developed for a student at school.

Special education teachers normally have additional training in working with students who have learning and emotional disabilities; these teachers can be sophisticated in their approaches to classroom behavioral problems. Mental health consultants and special education teachers make natural allies, sharing common ground in attempting to understand and deal with most disabled young people. Depending on background and interest, guidance counselors, often master's-level teachers with a school counseling degree, provide more in-depth services to students such as group work (social skills groups, divorce groups), promote schoolwide preventive programs (e.g., conflict resolution), and generally work to develop a more thorough understanding of individual students and their families. In the primary grades especially, many counselors work to help prevent and alleviate the behavioral or emotional problems of their pupils. School psychologists are trained at the master's or doctoral level and are knowledgeable about childhood psychopathology in the school setting. School psychologists may be responsible for many schools (mainly engaging in psychological testing for decisions about eligibility for special education) and may be less available for direct clinical interventions. School principals and assistant principals, successful individuals within the educational system, bring significant experience and knowledge about students and the educational system by virtue of their years in education. Their beliefs and attitudes about emotional disorders set the tone for the entire school. Senior school administrators can be powerful allies to the school mental health consultant.

▌ DEVELOPING A CONSULTATIVE RELATIONSHIP WITH SCHOOLS

Getting Started

Issues that aspiring school mental health consultants must consider before jumping into consultative work include their reasons for seeking to do school consultation (e.g., financial, political, or ethical objectives; personal and professional satisfaction) and a basic idea of what they intend to accomplish. Practically, they should be clear about the time they can commit to such work (i.e., clinical evaluations can be more time intensive than consultation). Other questions to consider before getting started include the following: Will I get paid for my work? What am I willing to do and not do as a consultant (i.e., how do I define my role concretely)? How will my role definition affect my negotiations with the school? Questions about role definition might include the following: What is my direct responsibility for students' welfare? Will I engage students' families during the course of the consultative work? Will consultation and education about mental health issues to school staff be conducted? Will direct student observation be part of the consultations even if direct evaluative services are not offered? Will lectures or seminars be proposed? What type of school (e.g., private vs. public; elementary vs. middle vs. high school; schools for handicapped, emotionally disturbed, special education, or learning disabled students; magnet schools for the gifted and talented) will I consult to? What staff will I interact with on a regular basis (e.g., principals, school psychologists, special education teachers, counselors)? Will I provide treatment services beyond simple evaluations at the school? The answers to these questions and others must be decided on and negotiated with the target school(s) before beginning consultative work. Consultants must be sensitive to and aware of each school's perceived mental health needs as well as their own consultative agenda when negotiating such work; the final agreement will likely reflect a mixture of the consultant's and the school's agendas.

School administrators may feel desperate for interventions and—especially at the outset—may be uncomfortable with simply receiving advice and recommendations that they have to implement themselves. The final answers to the questions above (and others) are normally determined through discussion with administrators of the particular school or school district with whom you make a consultative arrangement. Often the expected role of the consultant, at least initially, is to alleviate the problems encountered with particular students. This expectation is often manifested as the desire for the consultant to directly treat students and to take responsibility for these problem individuals. Unless the proper role of the consultant is clarified, the beginning of a new consultative relationship can be fraught with misunderstanding. The primary mission of school consultation must be emphasized to enhance the ability of administrators, teachers, and support staff to deal with the emotional or behavioral disturbances of students at school and to promote positive mental health throughout the school (Arnold et al. 1993).

Where and Whom to Approach

Given the broad array of schools with which to consult, gaining access to the local schools is a varied and individualized process. To begin the process of entering a school and establishing a professional relationship, a consultant must have sanction from the proper authority. Many principals have this authority; in some cases the authority is held by the central administration. Personal relationships go a long way toward gaining access to a school system. An introduction by a staff member of the school greatly enhances initial access. One simple approach is to build on existing relationships with teachers, principals, school counselors, school psychologists, and others in the community to obtain the needed introduction to the sanctioning authority. School counselors are often receptive to an unsolicited call offering a free lecture and letting them know of a consultant's interests. Such calls might also be made to special education teachers, to the central administration offices, or to the head of guidance counseling or special education in smaller school districts. These people may be able to arrange meetings with the principal and with other interested or involved school personnel to get the process under way.

When making unsolicited calls to gain access to a particular school or set of schools, the consultant should respect the hierarchy of the local school system. Consider the possibility that local school principals will react negatively if contact is initiated with their superiors to gain access to their school. The school principal must be aware of your intentions and interest before you arrive on school property. Even if principals delegate the authority for working with a consultant to a subordinate, they *must* be involved and informed about your activities.

Contacting other mental health professionals in the community who already engage in school consultation is another relatively simple way to tag along with their existing relationships. Local chapters of professional organizations such as the American Academy of Child and Adolescent Psychiatry, the National Association of Social Workers, the American Nurses Association, or the American Psychological Association will often have information about who is engaged in school consultation in the local community.

Further Negotiations

Because school staff often see the consultant as concrete help, your availability and role in relation to school personnel outside the agreed-on hours must be strictly established. It is very unsettling to be called at 4:00 P.M. on a Friday afternoon by a distressed principal with an agitated or suicidal student in her office. How you respond to crises, if called on, often constitutes a test of your abilities, usefulness, and commitment. Setting guidelines for such issues up front will prevent inevitable difficulty later in the relationship. The goal of a consultative relationship should be to increase the school's autonomy in managing mental health problems and not to increase the school's dependency. Existing services both within and outside the school and how to augment them should be considered when devising consultative arrangements.

Informed Consent

If the consultative contract (be it a handshake or a written agreement) includes the individual review of confidential student records or student interviews or observations, gaining informed consent from a student's family is critical. The need to gain consent should be discussed with the principal, and an arrangement should be made to obtain written consent if it is considered necessary. Obtaining actual consent is typically the school's responsibility. Various approaches to this issue can be taken. One very supportive principal sent all parents a consent form stating that mental health consultants were available to the school and requesting blanket consent for the consultant to evaluate any or all children and classrooms. Case-by-case written consent is another often-used method, usually implemented by the guidance counselor. Consultants who are official school employees during their hours of consultation may have a diminished need for written consent. In any case, the right of the child and the family to accept or refuse mental health care services must be respected.

Remuneration

Negotiations must also include what the school needs to provide in return (money, office space, telephone access, referrals) for the consultative services. Numerous types of formal arrangements may be constructed. In some, you may become a full- or part-time school district employee. Other arrangements include contracting on a fee-for-service basis for evaluation and treatment services, Medicaid billing if you are setting up a satellite clinic at a school, working under a state mental health block grant, or free consultation as a pro bono activity or to establish yourself within the community.

Delivering Consultative Services at Schools

The development and implementation of the consultant's plan within a school involves an amalgamation of the school's perceived needs, the available opportunities for consultation, and the consultant's perceptions of the needs of the school. Remuneration arrangements and decisions made during the negotiation process shape the consultant's activities. Even if direct, evaluative, school-based services are the main thrust of the consultative contract, programmatic consultative services often enter into discussion as individual student needs are addressed. The converse may be true, as recommendations regarding the needs of individual students may emerge from a discussion about making programmatic changes at the school.

Direct Evaluative Services

A comprehensive, streamlined format is essential for conducting school-based evaluations of students' psychiatric issues and needs. Mattison (1993) developed an excellent format for such evaluations. These evaluations should take advantage of the information provided by the school, information obtained from the family, and information acquired from classroom observation. This allows a relatively brief evaluation to have meaning. Recommendations must be school relevant. Recommendations regarding a student's eligibility for special education services or outside referral must be supported by clear clinical data. Working closely with the teacher, school psychologist, and guidance counselor in the course of evaluations and communicating respect for their ideas will increase the efficacy of your recommendations. The art of diplomacy is very important if it becomes necessary to contradict others' beliefs about what is best for a particular student. Support your position with clinical data that are easily understood by all and refrain from making blanket statements. Reach early agreement on important items within the clinical evaluation report: how it is generated, who sees it, and how it is to be delivered. The child and family have a right to confidentiality, period. In special education eligibility meetings, clarify your personal involvement and personally present your evaluation findings. The presentation of a typed report in a meeting without the consultant being present can greatly limit the overall impact of the consultation. Meeting with the family as part of the special education eligibility process and making recommendations are functions that you should not relinquish. It is most appropriate for you to personally communicate your findings as part of the educational team. The following example is a description of a pupil- or case-centered consultation:

> Karen, a pleasant 9-year-old fourth grader, was achieving relatively low grades despite her apparent intelligence, which was a cause for concern by her school counselor and teacher. Referral to the special education study committee had previously been denied because she was not a behavioral problem in class and her academic performance was considered to be on grade level. Discussions with her teacher and a review of what was known about her family—Karen's older brother had been treated for attention-deficit/hyperactivity disorder (ADHD)—revealed that Karen likely had the inattentive subtype of ADHD. With the support of the new school consultant, the counselor arranged a conference that included the teacher and the consultant. More information was gathered from the mother, and the consultant and counselor were able to persuade Karen's family to take her to an outside evaluator, who confirmed the diagnosis and successfully began stimulant therapy.
>
> The consultant continued to inquire about Karen's performance. It had improved, but Karen continued to show significant scatter in her abilities. Although the consultant was unable to convince the school to provide psycho-

logical testing, Karen's counselor suggested this to the family. Karen was diagnosed with a superior IQ, yet she demonstrated a 20-point spread (more than one standard deviation) between her verbal and her performance abilities. With the support of the consultant, Karen was eventually placed in a program for gifted/learning disabled students that had just been made available within the school district.

Programmatic and Indirect Services

A constant focus of the consultant should be to develop a positive and collaborative relationship with the school staff. An affable, relaxed, nonofficious approach to school relationships, in which you are clearly interested in understanding more about the school and the experience of school staff, will go far in enhancing the impact of the consultation. Consider offering to deliver talks to school staff or to participate in discussions with them about topics pertinent to child and adolescent mental health and development. Teachers and counselors often appreciate the opportunity to learn and to ask questions on topics pertinent to their particular situations. Participating regularly in special education eligibility meetings and providing input to IEPs can have a tremendous impact on individual students and can increase the knowledge base of the special education committee on mental health issues. The opportunity to work with a group of educators in a variety of formats regarding emotional and behavioral problems within the school is a valuable part of the consultative process. Examples of consultative efforts include participation in a teacher's group focusing on student mental health issues; consultation to the school principal or assistant principal about problematic children or programmatic issues; and meeting regularly with the school psychologist, social worker, or counselor (or any combination of these) to discuss current pupil problems and issues. You may also meet with regular classroom and special education teachers or in groups to discuss certain children, mental health topics, or classroom behavior management or to assist school counselors to lead parent skills training or parent support groups.

The variations and combinations of consultative arrangements are limited only by imagination and practicality; they depend on the perceived needs of the school, the direct versus the indirect method of service delivery, the school's goals in the use of mental health consultation, your goals for the consultation, and the particular school environment.

The next case example demonstrates how the nature of a case-centered consultation may expand to a consultee-centered problem:

As Karen's case progressed through the school year, the school guidance counselor, with whom the consultant worked closely, began to divulge personal aspects of her own life. The conversation during the consultative hour frequently turned to the counselor's own abuse as a child and her difficulties in maintaining nonabusive adult relationships. This situation began to make school visits uncomfortable for the consultant, who often felt forced into the role of therapist to the counselor and frequently tried to redirect the conversations back to student issues. Because this effort did not seem to alleviate the situation and because the consultant was fearful of cutting off a valuable ally within the school, the counselor's issues were reflected back into the consultative work in the form of observations and questions. For example, the consultant observed that the counselor had significant strengths in recognizing children who were quietly suffering such as Karen, but also gently noted her difficulty in feeling empathic with aggressive children and with parents she considered insensitive. As a result of these discussions and the renewed focus on the counselor's awareness of her own style and how it affected the identification and disposition of many students, the counselor opted to begin psychotherapy herself to enhance her self-understanding and her efficacy in her job.

A shift in consultation focus like the one described in this vignette must be enacted cautiously.

Necessary Skills of the Consultant

Besides the capacity to assess children from a biopsychosocial and developmental perspective, the school consultant must have a solid grasp of systems theory. Each student evaluated represents an individual child as well as a representative of two overlapping (and at times conflicting) systems: the family and the school. The consultant must be able to consider all related factors when making recommendations *that do not conflict with these overlapping systems.* Familiarity with the school system and the school in question is very important, yet a priori knowledge about the school is not essential. Most important is a sincere curiosity and a wish to learn about how the school functions and its strengths and weaknesses. A thorough understanding of the school will help the consultant make recommendations that are not outside the capacity of the school to implement. Although the personality characteristics of a successful school consultant are not written in stone, an open-minded approach to the foreign environment that the school represents, a desire to learn about the school and the experience of the personnel who work within it, an honest respect for fellow professionals, and an understanding and observance of the school hierarchy create a climate that aids the school in accepting an outsider. Being reflective yet practical, taking action to help without "de-skilling" school personnel, and observing the boundaries of your role are abilities that come with experience in consultation. An effective consultant continually keeps the balance of these competing tensions in mind when working in the schools.

Finally, readiness and willingness to enter into uncharted territory are vital. For example, supporting school administrators when a need is expressed—such as responding to a school suicide, an episode of violence, or another critical incident—will increase your skill and satisfaction and will cement the relationship with the school immeasurably.

Pitfalls and Problems

The role of consultant is complex and requires continual maintenance. Resistance from certain school personnel to a consultant's efforts or recommendations is a problem frequently cited by consultants. The consultant's "opponents" may have many reasons for their resistance. Staff members may feel uncomfortable or anxious in the presence of a mental health professional and may espouse a lack of support for or belief in mental health concepts in general. The consultant may be seen as a threat to the importance or authority of certain staff members within the school, who may feel devalued by virtue of the consultant's presence or attitude. The resistance may stem from negative past experiences with mental health services or a simple lack of experience. Regardless of the reasons for the conflict, your capacity to show an interest in the other's position and views without feeling offended or threatened by the resistance, in addition to the capability to exhibit gentle persistence in the face of adversity, will often determine the eventual success or failure of the consultative relationship.

Role confusion is the most insidious of all pitfalls for the consultant. Mental health consultants are trained to evaluate and often take primary responsibility for their patient. The role of the consultant is to carry out the primary mission previously stated and to support the school in remaining responsible for its students. Moving into the position of primary caretaker within the school setting is generally a violation of the consultative role. Maintaining the proper role while not appearing distant or uninvolved is the art of enhancing the relationship with the school.

The educational system is responsible for training and modifying the behavior of children in addition to teaching them in formal subjects. Out of this institution has emerged an entire lexicon of terms and concepts relating to the mental health problems of students within the schools. A major area of conflict between educators and mental health clinicians concerns the terms *emotional disorder* and *behavioral disorder*. Within many school systems, emotional disorders such as depression, anxiety, or psychosis are viewed as real conditions requiring special education services. On the other hand, behavioral problems may be seen as simple problems of discipline. This perspective can create conflict, because the clinician often feels that behavioral problems have emotional and neuropsychiatric roots and that students with such problems are equally deserving of special education services as those with emotional problems. School administrators may cite various laws requiring them to provide "appropriate" services, not the optimal services for which clinicians often strive. The final example touches on some of the pitfalls encountered in the context of a programmatic consultation:

> Through his participation on the special education eligibility committee, the consultant noted, near the end of the school year, a split within the school staff. The school counselor represented one faction, who felt that emotional disorders were being "swept under the carpet" by the school administration. The opposing faction expressed the view that schools were for educating children, not treating them. Despite education about mental health issues provided by the consultant at the eligibility meetings, strong disagreements surfaced. The consultant had attempted to support the school psychologist, who tried to moderate these open conflicts. Because of the concerns over the split, the consultant arranged a meeting with the school principal. The principal was caught between the demands for higher scores and a shrinking budget, so she admitted that she had little time to address the issues of a select few students in need of special education services.
>
> After the summer break, it was still unclear how this conflict might be addressed. The consultant was mindful of his role, because he realized that open advocacy for the needs of emotionally disabled students would certainly place him on one side of the conflict and minimize his effectiveness. The consultant continued to persevere in working with the guidance counselor and teachers regarding individual student problems. In midwinter, shocking news broke that an 11-year-old boy at the school had tried to hang himself. He had been noted to be quiet and an underachiever, yet he had not attracted any special attention. The faculty was greatly concerned, and, because of previous contacts with the principal, the consultant was asked to help facilitate meetings with faculty members about recognizing psychiatric disorders in children. These discussions were fruitful, and a prevention campaign, which included the parent-teacher organization, was developed to educate families and teachers about childhood mental disorders. Monthly meetings with the school principal were instituted to discuss school mental health issues and how they were related to good academic performance and program structure. A spin-off of this effort was aimed at strengthening the school–family working alliance, and a number of programmatic initiatives were carried out over the next 2 years.

Regardless of what you as the consultant feel is best, school personnel are free to disregard your input. Without your role firmly in place as a consultant, you can easily end up on one side of a conflict. Such polarization of the role renders a consultant less effective. In addition, legal and ethical concerns may arise in the course of consultation. These often involve issues of confidentiality and child safety. A consultant needs to ensure the safety and welfare of all children. If a child is being abused or is at risk of significant harm, the consultant must inform the proper individuals and institutions. The school principal is ultimately responsible for all children in the school and needs to be included in the consultant's concerns and plan.

▌ CONCLUSIONS

The essentials of school consultation can be summarized as follows:

- Develop an access point to the school or school system.
- Establish sanction for the consultative relationship to begin (or continue); this typically emanates from the school principal or central administration office.
- Establish the goals and purpose of the consultative efforts in collaboration with the sanctioning authority and interested stakeholders within the school (e.g., principal, vice principal, counselor, psychologist, special education teachers).
- Define the scope of the consultative work and the limits of your responsibility.
- Become familiar with the external forces and issues impinging on the school and develop a sense of the school's personality and the leadership styles within the school hierarchy.
- Get to know the various players (school staff) whom you will have regular contact with. Get a feeling for their roles within the school, their responsibilities, their areas of strength and weakness, and their personalities.
- Maintain an attitude of openness, curiosity, collegiality, and mutual respect at all times when dealing with school personnel.
- Regardless of the problem presented, make sure that any recommendations or plans that you make are practical, are at the skill level of the staff implementing them, and are felt to be relevant or useful by the school personnel.
- Maintain sight of the overarching goal of increasing the school's sophistication in managing mental health issues regarding its student body, thereby making the school more independent of your presence rather than dependent on it.
- Keep an eye open for opportunities to provide education and programmatic consultative services when appropriate and in a nonthreatening manner.
- Be patient and maintain the boundaries of your role as a consultant; it can take several years to establish a sophisticated and mutually rewarding consultative relationship.

▮ REFERENCES

Arnold LE, Ascherman LI, Belfer ML, et al: Psychiatric Consultation in Schools: A Report of the American Psychiatric Association. Washington, DC, American Psychiatric Association, 1993

Berlin IN: Mental health programs in the schools, in Child and Adolescent Psychiatry, Sociocultural and Community Psychiatry, 2nd Edition (American Handbook of Psychiatry Series, Vol 2). Edited by Caplan G. New York, Basic Books, 1974, pp 735–748

Caplan G, Caplan RB: Mental Health Consultation and Collaboration. San Francisco, CA, Jossey-Bass, 1993

Education for All Handicapped Children Act of 1975, Pub. L. No. 94-142

Education of the Handicapped Act of 1965, Pub. L. No. 89-313

Education of the Handicapped Act Amendments of 1986, Pub. L. No. 99-457

Education of the Handicapped Act Amendments of 1990, Pub. L. No. 101-476

Elementary and Secondary Education Act Amendments of 1965, Pub. L. No. 89-750

Mattison RE: A model for SED case evaluation, in Child and Adolescent Mental Health Consultation in Hospitals, Schools, and Courts. Edited by Fritz GK, Mattison RE, Nurcombe B, et al. Washington, DC, American Psychiatric Press, 1993, pp 109–129

APPENDIX
Brief Glossary of School Terminology

admission, review, and disposition (ARD)   Frequently used to describe committees of school personnel (e.g., teachers, special educators, administrators, school psychologists) and parents who meet to establish the eligibility of any given student for special education services and to ratify the proposed Individual Educational Plan (IEP) for that student.

emotionally disturbed (ED)   Shorthand for services pertaining to the emotionally handicapped.

Individual Educational Plan (IEP)   Describes the types and quantity of special education services a student will receive and the specific disabilities, skills, and target behaviors to be addressed during the course of service delivery. Updated at least yearly.

learning disabled (LD)   Shorthand for services pertaining to those with learning disabilities.

mentally retarded (MR)   Shorthand for services pertaining to the mentally retarded population.

other health impaired   Children found eligible for special education services who do not fall within the learning-disabled or emotionally disturbed categories (e.g., those with physical handicaps, chronic medical problems, human immunodeficiency virus [HIV] infection, and more recently, attention-deficit/hyperactivity disorder [ADHD]).

Public Law (P.L.)   Pertains generally to the Education for All Handicapped Children Act of 1975 (P.L. 94-142) and its subsequent amendments, which mandate a free and appropriate education to all students regardless of disability, from birth to age 21 years.

resource room   A classroom staffed by a special education teacher and possibly assistants to provide special education services to students for limited periods of time in a variety of subjects.

self-contained classroom   A special class with a low student-to-teacher ratio; used for more disabled students requiring more individualized attention and structure for academic progress.

special education   Generic term referring to the administrative and educational system mandated by public law to provide free and appropriate education to students who have intellectual, learning, emotional, or other health handicaps or disabilities.

11 SCHOOL-BASED HEALTH CENTERS

Mark D. Weist, Ph.D.

Laura A. Nabors, Ph.D.

Kathleen E. Albus, Ph.D.

Tanya N. Bryant, B.S.

National movements are under way to bring more comprehensive health care and mental health care to youths in schools (U.S. Public Health Service 2000; Weist et al. 2003a). Mental health programs in schools assume many forms. We use the term *expanded school mental health* (ESMH) to capture key elements of a full continuum of mental health promotion and intervention offered to youths in both regular and special education through partnerships between schools and other community systems (Weist 1997). A major impetus for the growth of ESMH programs nationally has been school-based health centers (SBHCs), which offer comprehensive physical and mental health care to students (Center for Health and Health Care in Schools 2001; Juszczak et al. 1995). As SBHCs have been established across the nation at more than 1,400 schools, support has been provided for ESMH programs, because mental health problems are the number one or number two reason for referral in most centers (Anglin et al. 1996; Center for Health and Health Care in Schools 2001). In Baltimore, Maryland, we have considerable experience in the development of ESMH programs and SBHCs, as well as in integrating these two approaches to health care (Weist et al. 2003b).

This chapter provides background about ESMH programs, particularly those connected to SBHCs. To illustrate issues encountered in these programs, throughout the chapter we convey experiences of our School Mental Health Program (SMHP), an ESMH program that is currently operating in 28 schools in Baltimore, with 8 of these schools having SBHCs.

■ UNIVERSITY OF MARYLAND SCHOOL MENTAL HEALTH PROGRAM

The SMHP of the University of Maryland Department of Psychiatry currently provides ESMH in 28 Baltimore City schools. The program's mission is to provide comprehensive and empirically supported services to youths in need in a proactive, energetic, and flexible manner. Because the number one attribute of ESMH programs is enhanced access to care, we strive to maintain high accessibility of our program to youths in need. This is exemplified by the fact that in the schools, clinicians often see 12 or more children in a day, compared with the 3–6 they see in community mental health centers (CMHCs). In this context, clinicians are able to observe and interact with youths in a variety of settings (e.g., office, hallway, cafeteria, gym, assembly) and consequently can gain a greater understanding of factors affecting the behaviors of the children and adolescents they serve.

Clinical services provided in our ESMH program are summarized in Table 11–1. These services include focused evaluation, diagnostic assessment, case management, a range of therapies, prevention and mental health promotion activities, and staff consultation. Interventions focus on issues that are endemic with inner-city youths from low-income families, who often face problems related to exposure to violence, abuse and neglect, bereavement, familial substance abuse, depression, anxiety, behavioral problems, and school performance issues.

TABLE 11–1.   Expanded school mental health: clinical services provided

---

Evaluation and diagnosis

Case management

Therapy

Prevention efforts

Mental health promotion

Consultation to school staff

Intervention for school-specific needs

Liaison to community resources

Staff training on mental health issues

Consistent with our mission, clinicians work collaboratively with the other mental health providers in the school (e.g., school social workers, psychologists, and guidance counselors) in schoolwide efforts to address pressing problems. For instance, our efforts include the development of crisis intervention plans for use after tragedies such as the violent death of a student (which in most of our schools occurs one or more times in a year). In addition, we act as a bridge for the school, helping to connect it and its students and staff to a full range of community resources and providing training to school staff on the early identification of youths who may need assistance (Flaherty and Weist 1999).

Consultation and Primary Care

A major issue for those interested in providing mental health services in the schools is addressing the question of whether consultation or primary care services will be provided. Mental health professionals have been working in the schools for a long time, and for some disciplines (e.g., child psychiatry) the major role has been providing consultation. In Baltimore, the funders have conveyed their preference for hands-on programs, with consultation a less desired service. However, this preference does not indicate that consultation is not valuable. Rather, a decision needs to be made about whether the program will be involved in hands-on delivery of clinical and preventive services, will provide consultation, or will do both. In our SMHP we chose to do both, with some staff members (e.g., clinical social workers, postdoctoral fellows in psychology) providing clinical services and other staff members (e.g., psychiatry and psychology faculty members, child psychiatry fellows) offering primarily supervisory and consultative services.

Pitfalls to Avoid Early On

Our experience has been that successful programs are characterized by leaders and by staff who keep the interests of children and adolescents in the forefront and are genuinely committed to participating in team efforts to improve services for them. In contrast, we have observed programs come and go on the school health scene in the city. Some of the major characteristics of school health programs that have not succeeded in Baltimore include 1) proceeding with traditional client service delivery models, such as providing only tertiary care and doing so fairly passively (e.g., bringing the CMHC into the school and waiting for the students to come); 2) operating from a bureaucratic or legalistic perspective, maintaining barriers to care (e.g., extensive screening procedures, lengthy intake processes), and referring many children out for services; 3) conveying clinical or professional superiority, which is often combined with a disinterest in other ideas and perspectives; 4) having veiled interests—for example, providing a façade of clinical interest when the real interest is gaining access to populations to conduct research; and 5) participating minimally (or not at all) in interagency committee work and planning.

We now turn to a more in-depth exploration of the nuts and bolts of our SMHP: from setting up referral mechanisms, to developing services, to implementing quality assurance and evaluation plans.

Establishing a Referral Base

Establishing close relationships between school mental health staff, other school personnel, and community organizations is critical to the success of the program for many reasons. When a program is beginning, it is usually important to conduct a number of presentations—for example, in classrooms, at staff meetings, and at parent-teacher association meetings—to describe the program and its benefits and to convey how to initiate a referral.

Referral sources for school mental health programs are many and varied. If the program is connected to an SBHC, most referrals will likely come from school health staff (e.g., nurses, nurse practitioners). These referrals will commonly be followed by referrals from teachers, other school mental health staff, school administrators, and students and families. If the program is not connected to an SBHC, referrals will mostly come from teachers and the other groups just mentioned. There are two major issues to attend to in establishing a referral base. First, it is important to do so in a way that promotes collaborative relationships with other staff in the school. Hence, it will be important to be responsive to the referral and to provide the referring person with feedback regarding the referral's status. Second, many school mental health staff members become inundated with a level of referrals they cannot realistically respond to. This underscores the need to maintain ongoing communication with all referring staff members to keep them up to date on one's ability to respond to new referrals.

Privacy, Confidentiality, and Ethical Issues

In schools in our program that are connected to SBHCs, consent for mental health services is included in the consent form to join the health center. We usually also contact parents to inform them that their child has been referred for services. Parents are invited to provide information during the intake process and are invited to join in the treatment process whenever possible. In high school, however, many adolescents do not wish their parents or families to be involved in treatment and are keenly interested in the therapy material remaining confidential. Despite this wish, we continually work with students to increase their receptiveness to family involvement in the sessions. For example, we usually emphasize to youths that the most effective help we can provide is to improve their situation *and* help them develop coping and problem-solving skills. Without family involvement, only the latter can be accomplished.

Several issues related to student privacy confront clinicians in schools. For example, students can be subjected to teasing if peers know that they are receiving therapy. Clinicians need to be sensitive to this matter. We work to reduce this potential stigma by providing anonymous passes (that do not list providers' names) for children to attend sessions at the health center. We also use the intercom to make anonymous calls into classrooms requesting a particular student to report to the main office. If we see our clients in the hallway, we try to be sensitive to their cues. In many cases we simply acknowledge students with a head nod or "hello" (without their names), and we respect their desire for interpersonal distance in public situations. Similarly, with students who are highly sensitive about privacy, we dismiss them from sessions during classes so they are not seen leaving the office by other students.

Mental health records are stored in a separate location from other health and school records. These records can be viewed only by members of the program staff, which is reassuring to youths and families but at times can be frustrating for those on the health and educational staffs. One approach to address this issue has been to release process information (e.g., whether a student has been attending sessions) but not content information (e.g., material discussed during therapy sessions) to certain staff members with the permission of the student. Because ESMH programs are developing, there are many areas where clear standards are not in place. One of these areas pertains to mental health records. In some programs these records belong to the SBHC; in other cases they belong to the school or to the collaborating CMHC. Our view has been that these records should be maintained separately to provide an additional degree of protection of confidentiality for students, because confidentiality is often hard to maintain in schools (Evans 1999). In addition, there is a real threat of long-term negative consequences for youths who receive mental health services (e.g., sharing of information by insurance companies, pejorative connotations of diagnoses, and denial of opportunities for military or federal service). Therefore, we believe that labeling youths as patients should be avoided unless they should clearly be part of the public mental health system (i.e., based on legitimate and concerning diagnosis and some level of risk). Maintaining separate records helps to protect against loss of confidentiality and against these longer-term risks.

Reducing the stigma of receiving mental health services is another critical issue facing ESMH programs. Youths usually have a limited idea—if any—of what a psychologist or psychiatrist does, and they often confuse the meaning of "social worker" with the role of a protective service worker. Thus, we identify ourselves simply as counselors or doctors. Although such generic language does not convey to students our specific roles or functions, it does prevent confusion and stigma associated with professional labels.

Therapy Services

Characteristics of therapy services provided are listed in Table 11–2. Individual, group, and family therapies are primary activities for clinicians. The duration of therapy can be short (one or two sessions) or long (a year or more). Most clinicians in our program approach therapy with a cognitive-behavioral orientation, but some dynamic methods are used, particularly with youths who have been traumatized (e.g., revisiting and expressing emotions from past abuse). We strive to ensure that all of our therapeutic interventions are developmentally appropriate and, whenever possible, based on evidence of positive impact (Weist 2003a).

We strive for cultural competence in all aspects of our program through specific training and by encouraging all staff members to learn about and immerse themselves in the school and the neighborhood. Staff members are encouraged to join in or initiate school and neighborhood work groups. For example, we are currently involved in a mentoring program through partnership with churches that surround program schools. Another good idea is for the program to have an advisory board including key stakeholder groups of youths, families, school staff, and community leaders, reflective of the racial and ethnic background of the community.

Youths are usually seen for individual or group sessions on a weekly basis. Sessions may be more or less frequent based on presenting problems. In individual sessions, students are typically seen for around 30 minutes. Keeping sessions shorter than an hour ensures that children will not miss too much classroom time. In an effort to initiate more controlled evaluation of our interventions, we have recently begun to use some manualized therapies for children and adolescents—for example, programs to address depression and impulsive behavior.

Group interventions vary for students in elementary, middle, and high school. At the elementary school level, groups focus on building behavioral and cognitive skills (e.g., self-control, problem solving, making friends). At the middle school and high school levels, groups are more process oriented, focusing on helping students cope and mutually support one another in relation to conditions of stress (including poverty; pervasive violence; and problems with school, family, and peers). In this context, we also teach skills and provide a forum for emotional expression related to past and current conflicts and traumas. Group sessions are usually longer than individual sessions, ranging from 45 minutes to an hour.

TABLE 11–2.   Expanded school mental health: characteristics of therapy services provided

Flexible duration
Largely cognitive-behavioral
Developmentally appropriate
Evidence based
Culturally competent
Representative of stakeholders' needs
Individual, family, and group sessions

Family Involvement

Family involvement is a challenge in ESMH, because in many schools it is very difficult to get families to come to the school to participate in therapy efforts. However, despite the challenge, we persist in trying to involve families as genuine collaborators in care because there is no doubt that when they are involved, assessments are more accurate and interventions are more powerful, as shown by numerous research studies (see Axelrod et al. 2003). Our work with families usually involves common elements of education (e.g., on common stressors and emotional/behavioral problems), training in behavior management, helping to improve communication with and supportiveness of youths, and generally helping the family and youth connect with school and community resources.

There is clearly an inverse relationship between the level of family involvement and school level, with the greatest degree of involvement occurring in our elementary schools, followed by middle schools. For high school students in our program, family involvement is limited in most cases and absent in some cases. Some teenagers in our program are highly resistant to their families being involved. These students often express concerns about confidentiality or fear of a negative reaction by a parent or guardian. Even in these cases, we make some effort to involve families. A frame that we sometimes use is that we are a neutral party who favors neither the teenager nor his or her parents and whose job is to enhance communication and mutual understanding, thereby bringing the adolescent and his or her parent or guardian closer together.

Working With Teachers and Other Staff

Providing services in schools affords unique opportunities for consultation and collaboration with teachers, clinicians from other disciplines, and school administrators. For example, the opportunity to observe children in various settings in an important natural environment is a critical advantage that, when taken, enhances the accuracy of the evaluation (Evans 1999). Also, working with teachers not only provides information about youths but also promotes teamwork with the teachers involving reciprocal training and complementary action.

Whenever possible, teachers should be invited to become a part of the school mental health team. These teacher leaders can assist the mental health staff in efforts to join with the school, for example, through presentations to the staff on mental health issues. Clinicians should approach these presentations with careful preparation and enthusiasm, because a group of 100 or more teachers tends to be a tough audience. For staff members who are uncomfortable with public speaking, relationships with the educational staff can be pursued individually and through small groups, such as committees.

We also work closely with school administrators. Having a close relationship with the school principal, which evolved from casual conversations held in the hallways, permitted one of our staff to petition for an in-school rather than an out-of-school suspension for a 16-year-old male student who had been fighting on school grounds. The staff member was able to share her observation that the teenager enjoyed being sent home during the day (as many adolescents would). When the consequences for fighting were changed to in-school suspension, during which the student worked with the school janitor on building maintenance, his disruptive behaviors decreased.

Case Management Services and Community Collaboration

Case management services are often critically important to the success of our efforts with students; however, activities such as arranging tutoring assistance, connecting a family with financial aid, or arranging for child care are often time-consuming. It can be a real challenge for clinicians to negotiate both therapy and case management demands. In an effort to ease these demands on clinicians, a number of support mechanisms have been put in place. These include close supervision, regular meetings of clinicians at the same school level (e.g., elementary school), sharing of successful strategies and ideas between staff members, and developing a support network in the school. Regarding the latter, we encourage clinicians to develop and maintain close relations with other school health and mental health professionals. These relationships often provide a source of support for clinicians when they are having difficulty arranging a needed resource for a student—for example, when we identify students who need assessment for special education services. Working closely with a school psychologist or social worker assigned to special education usually facilitates such a referral and at times helps to avoid an inappropriate referral.

Beyond such work with individual students, we encourage clinicians to join or help establish teams in the school. One example is the student support team, in which health and mental health providers from the school and community meet to coordinate activities and design special programs for youths, such as a schoolwide educational campaign on avoiding involvement in violence or on handling crises. Another example is the school improvement team, which coordinates broad schoolwide activities that focus on learning and on health and often involves the allocation of funds such as those provided through the Safe and Drug-Free Schools program. Through both teams, participants coordinate activities in the school and also seek to integrate school-based activities with broader initiatives occurring in the community.

We should also mention that as representatives of the public mental health system in the city, we have enhanced connections to community mental health programs, particularly those connected to our department of psychiatry. As such, we can serve liaison roles for the school in getting students who should be in the public mental health system to the appropriate service sites (e.g., CMHCs, psychiatric inpatient facilities, or residential programs). Our general rule is that students should be referred into the public mental health system when they present conditions of risk of harm to self or others, when there is some evidence of psychosis, or when there is an apparent need for medication. This advantage of facilitated connections to community mental health services for youths in need cannot be understated, because school personnel often express frustration about getting youths who need services in the community into those services. When difficulties are encountered in this process (as often happens), they can lead to inappropriate referrals into special education, because the staff may perceive that it is the only available option to address the student's problems.

Prevention and Mental Health Promotion Activities

Schools represent an ideal location to broadly promote student and family mental health and to prevent emotional and behavioral problems (see Graczyk et al. 2003). Our SMHP staff strive to serve as change agents (about 20% of their time), prevention specialists (about 50%), and clinicians (about 30%). The change agent role assists schools in improving the environment, for example, by establishing mentoring programs, ensuring a safe building, and introducing evidence-based life skills training into the curricula. To promote better use of the evidence base in child and adolescent mental health care, all staff members are trained to reduce stress and risk factors (e.g., exposure to violence, drug use), enhance protective factors (e.g., reading for pleasure, support from adults), teach validated skills (e.g., relaxation, self-control), and use manualized interventions (Weist 2002). The prevention role focuses on engaging in brief problem-solving interactions with youths and families, conducting skill-training groups, and carrying out collaborative work with educators to improve classroom behavior.

Program Evaluation and Quality Improvement

School mental health programs have been shown to improve school climate and reduce inappropriate referrals to special education (Bruns et al. 2003). Although there have been numerous studies of research-supported school mental health interventions, this research needs to expand in order to assess the impact of both ESMH programs and staff. Beyond such controlled research, programs can engage in other evaluation activities. For example, our program collects a range of measures evaluating clinical productivity (number of students seen, sessions held) and measures the services' impact on functional variables for individual students (grades, attendance, discipline encounters). These strategies document the productivity of the clinical staff and point to positive clinical impacts for many students.

In addition to individual student descriptive and outcome measures, ESMH programs should have a system of quality improvement, one of the most important activities for developing stable funding (Nabors et al. 2003). For measures reflecting program quality, we track staff training and supervision, educational presentations made in the school, and latency between referrals and first contacts with students. We ask students, teachers, and families to report what they like and do not like about our program and to report the efforts of individual staff members to improve services. A set of useful principles for best practice in ESMH has been developed by a national collaborative and may be a useful guide (Weist et al. 2005). Principles include an interdisciplinary staff, involved stakeholders, and evidence-based interventions.

Training Opportunities

Our program has a major focus on clinical training. Licensed clinicians in psychology and social work provide services and extend the person-hours and program outreach by supervising trainees and other clinicians. Affiliations with local graduate programs and the medical school for disciplines of clinical psychology, school psychology, counseling psychology, social work, psychiatry, and nursing are established through our department of psychiatry. Trainees attend our orientation program and monthly meetings that emphasize practical realities and effective strategies for working with inner-city youths in the schools. In 10 of our schools, fellows in child and adolescent psychiatry provide consultation for more intensive cases and collaborate with clinicians in prevention and mental health promotion activities. We strive to epitomize the collaborative model in which experienced staff, trainees, students, and families work together in a mutual problem-solving and supportive effort.

▌ CONCLUSIONS

Providing school mental health services in conjunction with an SBHC represents a multidimensional partnership including mental health, health, and education staffs working closely together and with important stakeholders of youths, families, and community leaders. Throughout the country, there are increasing calls for truly interdisciplinary efforts to improve health and mental health services for youths. We hope that our experiences, as reviewed in this chapter, capture the essence and the importance of this work.

▌ REFERENCES

Anglin TM, Naylor KE, Kaplan DW: Comprehensive school-based health care: high school students' use of medical, mental health, and substance abuse services. Pediatrics 97:318–331, 1996

Axelrod J, Lever NA, Ambrose MG, et al: Partnering with families in expanded school mental health programs, in Handbook of School Mental Health: Advancing Practice and Research. Edited by Weist MD, Evans SW, Lever NA. New York, Kluwer Academic/Plenum, 2003, pp 135–148

Bruns EJ, Walrath C, Glass-Siegel M, et al: Mobilizing research to inform a school mental health initiative: Baltimore's School Mental Health Outcomes Group, in Handbook of School Mental Health: Advancing Practice and Research. Edited by Weist MD, Evans SW, Lever NA. New York, Kluwer Academic/Plenum, 2003, pp 61–72

Center for Health and Health Care in Schools: School-Based Health Centers: Results From a 50-State Survey: School Year 1999–2000. Washington, DC, Center for Health and Health Care in Schools, 2001. Available at: http://www.healthinschools.org/sbhcs/survey2000.htm. Accessed February 6, 2005

Evans SW: Mental health services in schools: utilization, effectiveness, and consent. Clin Psychol Rev 19:165–178, 1999

Flaherty LT, Weist MD: School-based mental health services: the Baltimore models. Psychol Sch 36:379–389, 1999

Graczyk PA, Domitrovich CE, Zins JE: Facilitating the implementation of evidence-based prevention and mental health promotion in schools, in Handbook of School Mental Health: Advancing Practice and Research. Edited by Weist MD, Evans SW, Lever NA. New York, Kluwer Academic/Plenum, 2003, pp 301–318

Juszczak L, Fisher M, Lear JG, et al: Back to school: training opportunities in school-based health centers. J Dev Behav Pediatr 16:101–104, 1995

Nabors LA, Lehmkuhl HD, Weist MD: Continuous quality improvement and evaluation of expanded school mental health programs, in Handbook of School Mental Health: Advancing Practice and Research. Edited by Weist MD, Evans SW, Lever NA. New York, Kluwer Academic/Plenum, 2003, pp 275–284

U.S. Public Health Service: Report on the Surgeon General's Conference on Children's Mental Health: A National Action Agenda. Washington, DC, U.S. Government Printing Office, 2000

Weist MD: Expanded school mental health services: a national movement in progress, in Advances in Clinical Child Psychology, Vol 19. Edited by Ollendick TH, Prinz RJ. New York, Plenum, 1997, pp 319–352

Weist MD: Challenges and opportunities in moving toward a public health approach in school mental health. J Sch Psychol 41:77–82, 2002

Weist MD, Evans SW, Lever NA: Advancing mental health practice and research in schools, in Handbook of School Mental Health: Advancing Practice and Research. Edited by Weist MD, Evans SW, Lever NA. New York, Kluwer Academic/Plenum, 2003a, pp 1–8

Weist MD, Goldstein J, Morris L, et al: Integrating expanded school mental health programs and school-based health centers. Psychol Sch 15:297–308, 2003b

Weist MD, Sander MA, Walrath C, et al: Developing principles for best practice in expanded school mental health. J Youth Adolescence 34:7–13, 2005

12 FOSTER CARE PROGRAMS

Frances S. Porter, A.C.S.W., L.C.S.W.

Charles Huffine, M.D.

The primary traumas for children in foster care are the separation from and loss of their biological family added to the trauma from abuse and neglect that these children have experienced. To effectively provide treatment, mental health care providers need to understand the troubled backgrounds and subsequent emotional challenges of children in foster care. In this chapter, we present a historical perspective (illustrated in Figure 12–1) and discuss implications for mental health care providers working in the area of foster care.

▌ HISTORICAL PERSPECTIVE

Among the conclusions reached by the First White House Conference on the Care of Dependent Children, held in 1909, was that children without families were best placed in the community with substitute families instead of in orphanages. Awareness of the battered child syndrome in the 1960s led state agencies to investigate child abuse. Foster care first began as a voluntary system to support overwhelmed mothers; however, increased reports of child abuse and the prominence of abuse investigations changed foster care into a largely involuntary system. Long-term removal of children from families led to passage of the Adoption Assistance and Child Welfare Act of 1980 (P.L. 96-272). Federal funding led to growth in public- and private-sector child welfare agencies.

Child protective services units were established to investigate allegations of child abuse and neglect. Child welfare services struggled to find and license sufficient foster homes to meet the demand. In many states, the social service system developed special group homes and residential treatment programs to deal with children entering the system with severe emotional and behavioral problems. Private agencies supplemented state services and provided leadership for the emerging social service challenges. Universities developed research and service programs addressing the problems of abused and neglected children. The social service system, including private and academic contractors, has been called the de facto child mental health system because it must address the mental health aspects of issues relating to abused and neglected children. Child protective services agencies have variable relationships with family courts and with law enforcement and mental health system agencies that address the needs of children in foster care. Coordination of services between child-serving agencies and continuity of medical and psychiatric care emerged as daunting problems for foster care children. The publication of *Unclaimed Children* by Knitzer in 1982 led to a series of well-described developments (Pumariega and Winters 2003).

Problems with the social service system workforce increased as the system grew. Many social service system agency staff members with bachelor's degrees in human services fields are unprepared to understand and provide for the enormous needs of their clientele. Chronic funding problems with impossible case loads, overwhelming case problems, and inadequate supervision and consultation cause many state caseworkers either to burn out or to grow in their ability to deal with crises and mobilize resources. There is constant tension between idealistic inclinations and administrative realities, including unclear limits on who can be served and what can be done.

▍ PERMANENCY PLANNING

The Adoption Assistance and Child Welfare Act of 1980 (P.L. 96-272), enacted in response to problems of foster care children not returning home, set principles that remain the structural framework for permanency planning in the social service system: 1) maintain children in their own homes if possible, 2) return a placed child home to his or her biological family, 3) permit adoption, and 4) provide for long-term foster care. To keep children in their own homes, families were to receive early, intense, home-based services provided by a child welfare agency or a mental health care provider. The family preservation model of intensive, time-limited services assumes aggressive outreach and prevents foster care placement. During the time of this initiative, many effective, innovative countrywide programs emerged but were often seen as being too little, too late.

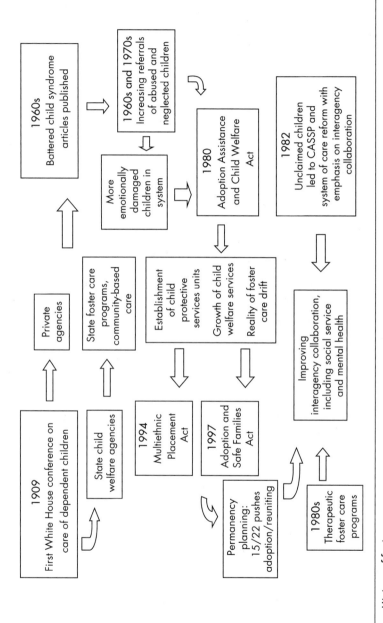

FIGURE 12–1. History of foster care.

CASSP=Child and Adolescent Service System Program.

If interventions fail, abused and neglected children must move from their biological family and be placed out of home, usually in foster care. More problematic children often go to group homes or residential treatment; children who are more difficult to place go to psychiatric hospitals or longer-term, more intensive residential programs. Some must leave home to be held in juvenile correctional institutions because of their own offending. Similar placements for equivalent problems in the justice system, rather than in the foster care or mental health care system, occur to a disproportionate number of minority youths. A child going into an out-of-home placement must have a judicial hearing in which the child welfare agency seeks custody of the child. After a child leaves his or her home, the emphasis is on rehabilitating the biological parents and having the child return home as quickly as possible. If this rehabilitation is not possible, the family and state personnel must return to court to decide either to immediately reunify the child with the family or to extend state custody.

Caseworkers are charged with the overwhelming task of helping children adjust to foster care; helping foster families understand and meet the foster child's needs; and providing case management services to promote birth parents' rehabilitation, including housing or employment resources, medical and mental health services, parenting education, and substance abuse counseling. The caseworker is responsible for facilitating parent–child visitations to assess appropriate interactions and the parents' understanding of their child's development. If the biological parents respond to these interventions, acknowledge some responsibility for their child's abuse or neglect, and integrate safe and healthy methods of parenting, their child is usually returned. Postreunification services must be provided for several months. If the reunification is successful, custody (or guardianship) is returned and the case is closed. Some parents of reunified families again abuse or neglect their children or acknowledge extreme difficulty in parenting their newly reunited children. Some children are never reunified because the parents are unable to become rehabilitated in the prescribed time. Then the agency attempts another permanency plan, usually adoption (or, rarely, long-term foster care with guardianship). In court hearings, the state must demonstrate that the family was provided adequate resources to enable them to rehabilitate, that the foster home was reasonably accessible to the biological parents, and that regular visits between parents and child were facilitated. The parents must demonstrate that they used the resources recommended by their caseworker, cooperated with community providers, and had regular visits with their child; they must also demonstrate that they are able to keep the child safe and will not abuse or neglect the child. An attorney or a guardian ad litem represents the child's legal interests. Foster parents have minimal or no standing in this legal process. Court stipulations may not seem to fit with the realities of parents' struggles to reclaim their children or the contracted agency's capabilities to provide services.

Some children continue in foster care despite little progress being made, with extensions of foster care and confusing arrays of poorly coordinated services, whereas other children are reunified prematurely. Rarely are services guided by best practice, based on research, and carefully coordinated between human service agencies. Daunting social problems beyond the scope of the social service system (e.g., parents being unemployed, having unsafe housing, or having their own serious mental health or substance abuse problems) are seldom addressed. Caught in impossible binds between the permanency needs of foster care children and the hope that their families will transcend the barriers to provide a safe and stable living environment, caseworkers must often face foster care children plaintively asking (despite their being at severe risk for further abuse), "When can I go home?" Children's lives can be affected by the dilemmas of permanency planning, as illustrated by the following example:

> Emilio, age 4 when entering foster care, followed five older siblings into foster care due to his mother's neglect. The court expected the mother to receive therapy, learn about parenting, and visit Emilio regularly. Intellectually limited and depressed, she made little progress in rehabilitation but was seen as nice. Emilio was placed in several foster homes, then in long-term foster care at age 8. When Emilio reached age 12, his foster parents wanted to adopt him. However, the court and welfare agency did not want to terminate parental rights. At age 14, able to care for himself with less parental supervision, he went home. The neglect cycle recurred; he returned to foster care within 2 years, but the foster family was no longer available.

In this case, adoption did not occur because the mother met minimum expectations.

States' initial efforts to enact programs based on permanency planning goals markedly reduced the numbers of children in foster care and seemed to be working until the late 1980s, when inadequate resources for children and biological parents extended the time some biological parents needed to rehabilitate. Time-consuming complexities in the adoption process surfaced. Long-term foster care has lacked support from most state administrators due to the expense of supporting a youth to adulthood. Some children stay in foster care for years, but policy prevents them from settling into foster homes where they are comfortable.

Increasing referrals of abused and neglected children led to high case loads of ever more difficult children and an atmosphere of pervasive crises and emergencies. Acute placements diluted the focus on adoption and long-term care. Permanency planning requires a well-developed, systematically executed plan within a prescribed time frame. Turnover in caseworkers, inexperience, and absent follow-through were added barriers to adoption or guardianship-based long-term foster care when return to birth families was unrealistic. Rising poverty, substance abuse, incarcerations, unemployment, homelessness, and human immunodeficiency virus (HIV) infection worsened the situation. Two pieces of federal legislation addressed the complex dynamics. The Multiethnic Placement Act of 1994 (P.L. 103-382) prohibits delay or denial of foster care or adoption placement solely on the basis of race, color, or national origin. Its impact is unknown. The Adoption and Safe Families Act of 1997 (ASFA; P.L. 105-89) prescribes aggressive promotion of legal permanency for foster care children through child welfare policy reform. ASFA emphasizes shorter, stricter time frames for birth parent rehabilitation, leading to family reunification and state financial incentives for case progression. Concurrent planning for reunification and for termination of parental rights leading to adoption is mandatory. The law's 15/22 rule mandates that states move for termination of parental rights when children have been in foster care for 15 of the previous 22 months unless "compelling reasons" for not pursuing termination can be documented. As states met the ASFA expectations, the dramatic increase in numbers of children freed for adoption put pressure on foster parents to adopt the children they were parenting when reunification efforts failed.

Daunting problems persist. Many children who need a permanent plan are in middle childhood or adolescence, have experienced trauma and disruptions, and are at high risk for mental illness. If foster parents do not adopt, then the child must again sustain disruption through adoption into another family. These adopted children remain at risk for more out-of-home or psychiatric hospital care. Although they have been abused, many enter adolescence yearning to reunite with their birth families. Experiencing drift from one placement to the next, they learn never to become fully attached, have difficulty establishing a relationship in their adoptive homes, and are at risk for disrupted adoption or for running away and living on the streets (Barth and Berry 1994).

It is too early to evaluate the impact of ASFA. Many youths who require foster care and adoption present with challenging behavioral and emotional difficulties. Adoption support programs funded through ASFA amendments help adoptive families acquire necessary services, but state commitment to such supports wanes in times of budget difficulties. Model programs have proved to be effective (e.g., Casey Family Services' Post-Adoption Services Program). Information on the adoption stability of former foster care children is scarce. Adoption disruption data are not systematically collected; estimates of failures depend on the population studied. Adoption is inappropriate for many adolescents; that is, permanency in adolescents is better defined in terms of enduring relationships with safe and significant adults, including relatives from the youth's birth family, rather than in terms of residential placement. In some social service and mental health programs serving older foster care children, the importance of the children maintaining relationships with siblings, cousins, or peers with whom they have had significant ongoing relationships is recognized. Stabilized placements for adolescents can range from guardianship arrangements in long-term foster care, to formal or informal kinship care, to informal board and care arrangements. An evaluation survey of informal programs in Seattle, Washington, produced an estimate that 48% of homeless youths were runaways from foster care or adoptive homes. The progression through foster care is illustrated in Figure 12–2.

▌ FOSTER CHILDREN AND FOSTER FAMILIES

Foster Children

Foster care children present with such complex problems that the welfare community must struggle to meet their needs. Frequently emerging in a child's story is a chaotic lifestyle involving multiple caretakers; moves into and out of other people's homes; and lack of predictable meals, sleeping times, or routines. School attendance is usually inconsistent. The child may have been in multiple school settings, had inadequate medical care, and witnessed substance abuse or domestic violence. Many foster care children have experienced physical or sexual abuse by adult caretakers, older siblings, or peers. Many do not know their father's identity and are often punished, rejected, or abused by their mother's various male friends. The oldest child may often be "parentified"—yearning to be grown up to be able to care for the entire family, including the mother, who is seen as helpless and in need of protection. Such children, who are at high risk for a host of medical and psychiatric problems, often have poor nutrition, frequent injuries, and neglected medical problems. Hidden problems in this population are the intellectual and mental health problems of fetal alcohol syndrome, cocaine exposure, and a panoply of other disorders (Carmichael-Olson et al. 1998). These children seldom see foster care as desirable. Separation, loss, grieving for their family, and dreaming of or waiting until they can go home are overriding issues affecting their adjustment to foster care and their developmental success. Mental health professionals must realize that many children feel guilty and disloyal for being reported as an abused and neglected child. Professionals must also be aware that conflicts and dysfunctional thinking can occur after a child is removed from the home when siblings remain (or are returned home after being placed in foster care). Most foster care children learn to be

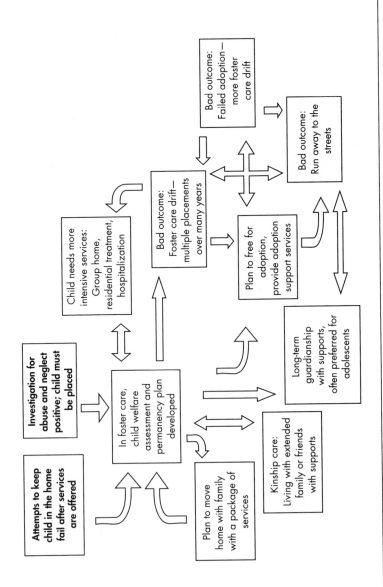

FIGURE 12–2. Progression through foster care.

survivors and become hypervigilant. Foster children often consider adults to be unreliable and potentially dangerous and relate to adults by saying what they think the adults want to hear. Although these children often seem older than their chronological age, they are usually emotionally underdeveloped:

> Tanya, an attractive 13-year-old girl, loved clothes and had the poise and verbal skills of a 16-year-old. As a child she lived with multiple "friends" of her mother; several of them sexually abused her. Placed in foster care after 6 years of residential treatment, she initially acted her age. Feeling more comfortable sitting between her foster parents and reading, talking, or watching television, she began to sit closer and closer to her foster mother, eventually inching herself onto her foster mother's lap. The foster parents were upset with this confusing behavior. The caseworker educated them about the impact of child sexual abuse and about pseudomaturity as an indicator of and response to victimization and trauma. The caseworker helped the foster parents understand that Tanya, emotionally younger, needed closeness and nurturance, and helped them accept this behavior by putting time frames and boundaries on it and making it "talkable" within the family. Tanya eventually gave up this behavior and demonstrated appropriate parent–child interactions.

Children often express distress behaviorally because they lack cognitive skills for verbally communicating feelings. Distressed foster care children may be cautious and polite verbally but demonstrate apparently incongruous behavior such as lying, stealing, hoarding, bed-wetting, throwing temper tantrums, fighting, running away, and withdrawing. A multidisciplinary team relationship with the foster or adoptive parent can usually deal with the expected deterioration in behavior when the child begins acting up or running away, which can occur when the child is incapable of responding to nurturance, reciprocity, and closeness (Table 12–1).

Foster Families

Foster parents are a very special group. Most have a love of children and seek to fulfill some ideal of being of service. They come from every walk of life, level of sophistication, marital status, age, and sexual orientation. Some have limited capacities to understand or tolerate the problems common to foster care children; others seem able to absorb with humor and good spirit anything a child presents. There is a severe lack of foster parents, and recruitment is difficult. When one delves beyond the idealism, motivations for becoming a foster parent seem to be mixed. Some become foster parents to assume a major rehabilitative role in the lives of children and run small virtual group homes. Some gravitate toward programs that train them to be part of the treatment team and to get support from clinical leaders in therapeutic foster care programs. Others become licensed to formalize an already existing living

TABLE 12–1.   The complex problems of foster children

Travails of foster children	Resilience factors for good outcomes
Hurt from abuse and neglect	Ability to form attachments with foster parents
Hurt from loss of family	
Hurt from role disruption with siblings	Being nurtured by contact with birth family
Inability to trust adults who care for them	
Susceptibility to psychiatric disorders	Remaining placed with or close to siblings
Predisposition to failure at school	Ability to commit to and function in school
Susceptibility to fetal damage from alcohol, cocaine, and malnutrition	Absence of symptoms of posttraumatic stress disorder, fetal damage, or mental illness
Alienation from culture and kin	
Difficulty forming an identity	Possessing an easy connection to culture and kin

situation (e.g., after becoming attached to a needy child who is a neighbor or a friend of their birth child). Those successful in this difficult role tend to be unique in their patience, tenacity, and commitment to their foster care children, making it through bad moments with faith that things will improve. Uniquely capable of seeing the child's strengths despite outrageous behavior, they have an instinct for defining needs. They do not personalize emotional assaults from the foster children or from a sometimes insensitive social service system. They become system wise and effective advocates for foster children in their care by being articulate in communicating children's needs in collaboration with professionals. Positive and negative attributes of foster parents are summarized in Table 12–2.

Foster parents are subject to confusing rules from sponsoring agencies. Orientations and periodic state training programs vary in quality and relevance, as does caseworker support. Few state and private agencies excel at preparing foster parents, which causes many to burn out and give up. Others fall into traps and act toward their foster children in ways that are questioned by the caseworker. Some are investigated for child abuse. Because tragic situations of abuse by foster parents have received excessive coverage in the media, foster parents as a group are treated with suspicion by state leaders reacting to the potential for lawsuits. Allegations of abuse by foster parents seem to be earnestly investigated, with foster parents being held to high standards of behavior. Subject to such scrutiny, foster parents often feel insulted and dispirited. Even without any allegation being made against them, many leave foster care service because they perceive themselves as being at risk. Rarely will a foster parent have a preexisting problem that leads him or her

TABLE 12–2.   Assets and liabilities of foster parents

Assets	Liabilities
Undying idealism	Having unrealistic expectations of foster children
Commitment to a child	
Being undaunted by impossible situations	Being easily caught by a foster child's projection of birth-family issues
Capability not to take things personally	
Capacity to find practical solutions to problems	Vulnerability to false allegations
	Getting caught up in reactions to the child's problems
Ability to understand and cope with an imperfect system	
	Negativity to disapproval by family and friends
A good support network of their own	
Ability to use supervision by caseworker well	Potential for problems from their own birth children
Capability to utilize support organizations for foster parents	

to child abuse. More commonly, problematic parenting occurs as the relationship with the foster child evolves in such a way that the child begins to evoke similar feelings in the new set of parents as those that existed in the child's birth family. This countertransference-like reaction is invariably misunderstood by the caseworker or foster parent, and certainly by those charged with investigating abuse allegations. Foster parents in such circumstances blame the caseworker, develop an overwhelmingly negative reaction to the child, and demand that the child be instantly removed, while feeling terrible about the situation and horrible about themselves. Holding foster parents accountable in a legalistic process for errors in parenting commonly leads to the loss of a foster home. These disasters can usually be avoided through adequate caseworker support and clinical consultation. In response to the increasingly difficult legal climate for foster parents, a support group, the National Foster Parent Coalition for Allegation Reform, was formed. The organization's Web site (http://members.aol.com/nfpcar) and that of the National Foster Parent Association (http://www.nfpainc.org) contain links to myriad state organizations that address such issues locally.

Foster parents are subject to criminal checks and intrusions into their personal lives when they are being licensed. Family issues become public as their functioning is reviewed by caseworkers and others involved in the team supporting the foster children. Many people become foster parents despite objections from family members and friends. These people must counter the community stigma regarding foster care children and their families. Dealing with birth families can be an ordeal for foster parents if the birth families are disruptive and intrusive and if support from the social service system is inadequate. Foster parents who have birth children at home have unique challenges to consider; their own children may be ambivalent about sharing their parents because they feel they have no voice in the decision, lest they displease their parents. The responses of the biological children must be considered. Even when the family works out the struggles in these new domestic relationships, biological children have to adjust to awkward or embarrassing situations that may occur in school or in the neighborhood:

> Donna was a complex 6-year-old whose early traumatic history was unknown. At times she reported auditory and visual hallucinations with signs of paranoia. In her specialized foster home, at school, and in the community she required a precise, consistent, and identical routine and verbal cues from all adult caretakers. She experienced terror if left alone for too long or exposed to slight changes in routine, had explosive temper tantrums, ran out into the street, acquired knives, stole, and frequently masturbated at home and school. The episodic behaviors disturbed and embarrassed the foster parents' biological children, ages 12 and 14, but they managed to accept Donna, who was generally sweet, pleasant, shy, and friendly. The ultimate stressor occurred when Donna started to masturbate in church and could not be distracted. Efforts to stop this behavior were unsuccessful until the foster mother had her family and friends sit in the pews surrounding Donna to give her the exact same gestures and verbal cues when she began to masturbate. The behavior was extinguished. Eventually Donna joined the church choir, and the biological children were proud to sing with her.

The biological children of foster parents can learn to accept living with troubled foster siblings. Many such children become foster parents as adults. Foster parents naturally become attached to children in their home and are joyful when the children reciprocate. However, foster parents must frequently endure the sadness of not having their love returned by a child with attachment problems and must cope with having little say in the outcome of the case. They develop opinions about the impact of visits by the birth parents on the emotional health of the child. These opinions can be shared with the caseworker, but such observations and opinions have no legal status. The role of foster parent is inherently difficult. It is an enormous gift to the community that so many families and individuals agree to take on this role and stay with it over many years.

Numerous attempts have been made to reform the disincentives facing foster parents and to offer them a more respected role in teams addressing the child's many service needs (e.g., the system of care reform movement). Foster families with long-term commitments to the children they raise are psychologically identified as the parents and become central to teams that plan for a wraparound process. The most directly empowering reform for foster parents is the movement toward therapeutic foster care (TFC). These programs are based on recognizing foster parents' knowledge of the child, making them part of the team to define a treatment plan, and providing special access to clinical consultation and support. This foster parent mobilization is best defined in well-researched TFC programs. The Foster Family–Based Treatment Association (FFTA), a national organization, identifies researched and recognized best-practice TFC that addresses the mental health needs of foster care children. The FFTA maintains a Web site (http://www.ffta.org) with links to such programs—for example, the well-researched Multidimensional Therapeutic Foster Care program of the Oregon Social Learning Center; the TFC program of the Amherst H. Wilder Foundation in St. Paul, Minnesota; and the United Methodist Family Services programs in Virginia. These programs are defined by time-limited care to address problems with foster children and birth families and aim to reunite families. Less formally researched programs can be found by searching the Web for TFC.

❚ IMPLICATIONS FOR MENTAL HEALTH CARE PROVIDERS

The complexity of the foster care system and the extreme needs of many foster care children create a difficult service delivery situation for mental health care providers. Especially for traumatized children, mental health care providers must be clear about their particular duties in a given role in the social service system and whether those duties are realistic and within their ability to offer. (For example, mental health care providers know that conducting a forensic examination with a foster child and his or her family precludes offering that child treatment services. Providing consultation to the staff of a program would preclude conducting a review of a family grievance regarding that program's services.) An accepted role in the foster care system must have clear limits; any expansion of the role should be done with careful analysis of the implications. On occasion, taking a child into one's private practice on referral from an agency with which one consults could be considered a conflict of interest; in other situations, it could be considered an example of superbly coordinated care. There are three primary categories of mental health service roles: forensic, consultative, and direct services.

Forensic Services

Many mental health care providers are asked to conduct evaluations of children to guide the social service agency in its legal responsibility to advise the court regarding custody or deprivation of parental rights. Such evaluations contribute greatly toward answering certain questions that are important under the law and toward integrating legal requirements with the needs of the child or family. In the forensic arena, it is best to know the players and their roles and to make clear decisions about how best to relate to each. A caseworker may ask for a full evaluation of the child or parent and request that specific questions be addressed. Such questions are best articulated by lawyers who understand the legal issues. In requesting a full evaluation, it is important to have an agreement from all involved attorneys that the report will be respected. In this model the court is the client, and the report addressing specific legal questions becomes evidence for the court to use in its determinations. The mental health care provider must not be identified as an agent for any of the parties involved. Participation in such evaluations may preclude consultative or treatment roles within the system.

A full evaluation involves interviewing all parties and integrating data as a formal evaluation report. This differs from an evaluation to meet the caseworker's needs or one conducted before initiating treatment. A brief evaluation of a child or a conversation with a foster mother documented in agency notes may be requested in a legal process. Should the mental health care provider be called to testify in such a case, the court will be informed that the provider has not conducted a full evaluation and cannot responsibly address the tough legal questions of concern.

Consultation

Although roles for mental health care providers as consultants are formally defined in few social service system agencies, in many such agencies that deal with disturbed children, regular consultation is considered essential:

> A small agency had several TFC children whose medication evaluation needs and follow-up were provided by many community physicians. Families and caseworkers were troubled about the types and dosages of medications prescribed, perfunctory follow-up by some physicians, and difficulty reaching providers. The agency approached a child psychiatrist about establishing a collaborative relationship in which assessment and follow-up would be provided by his practice. He agreed and provided timely, appropriate services that garnered him respect and admiration. Staff members and foster families appreciated his manner of talking to them in easy-to-understand language. When agency staff needed consultations, his services were quickly requested. He now meets biweekly with the staff, provides consultation, and offers leadership to treatment team meetings with foster parents.

The role and process of consultation are detailed in Chapter 1, "Working Within Communities." Direct service may be compatible with a consultative role; one enhances the other. Expanded roles (e.g., training for staff or foster parents on specific topics and later consultations on staff or administrative issues) may be natural extensions. Involvement in internal agency politics can be hazardous, but if handled sensitively, such involvement can markedly aid the organization.

Direct Services

Many mental health care providers find providing evaluation and treatment services for foster care children to be frustrating and nongratifying (Rosenfeld et al. 1998). Disruptions in foster care and sudden moves make follow-through with treatment plans precarious (e.g., patients are lost to follow-up; reestablishment of care is hampered by barriers to locating the child and arranging transportation given time constraints; difficulties in obtaining records of prior treatment or passing records on to new providers are magnified by new regulations). Many providers give up. Tragic cases in which medical needs of children were neglected due to inadequate information sharing have led to serious illness, death, lawsuits, and atrocious publicity for state agencies. Office-based practitioners contracting to see foster care children are often unfamiliar with the state's public mental health system (and many such systems are beset with severe budget problems, draconian managed care rules, and low reimbursement rates). To obtain services in some states, foster care children must be enrolled in a Medicaid program and public clinics. Many public mental health programs are grossly inadequate in service provision and are poorly coordinated with other services. Private foster care agencies may be able to fund private practitioners, but they too are limited by fiscal realities and the need for accountability.

Exemplary attempts at service provision have been made (Fine 1993; Gallagher et al. 1995; Kates et al. 1991; Pilowsky 1992; Rosenfeld and Wasserman 1990; Steinhauser 1991). Former foster care children give mixed reviews about the helpfulness of treatment services. Many view former therapists as irrelevant or at worst adversarial. Former foster care children report passively withdrawing in treatment, actively seeking to leave treatment through outrageous behavior, or even disrupting their placement. Helpful treatment was credited to the therapist's forming a close and stable relationship with the foster care children. Successful therapists acknowledge foster children's mix of feelings about family, losses they have incurred, and attachment difficulties they are experiencing in their current life and appreciate the barriers to dealing with these feelings in a clinical setting. In such circumstances, a therapist must become relevant to the children on their terms, serve as an advocate, and help them define their relationship with their foster or adoptive family. A foster care child may spend time anticipating being reunited with his or her birth family even if it will not occur until the youth's eighteenth birthday. Therapists provide developmental support by helping the youth deal with peer relationships, school, or jobs, rather than focusing on family issues.

Innovative services attempt interventions that are more contextually grounded than standard care. TFC services are planned and delivered by a team that is ideally multidisciplinary and includes foster parents. Key components for helping foster care children work through their trauma-based and developmental issues are collaboration and open communication between team members, particularly foster parents. Team members share their assessments of the child's strengths, difficulties, and needed interventions and respect everyone's contribution. Therapeutic moments are not the sole province of a mental health therapist but exist for anyone working with the child. Senior clinicians provide training and support and review how the team has followed the treatment plan and the impact the plan has on the child. Successful implementation requires all team members to see themselves as equal partners with different perspectives of the child based on their relationship, training, and education.

System-of-care programs that use a wraparound process view the concept of teams a bit differently. Families are respected as the center of what is termed a child and family team (CFT). Family is defined from a child's perspective. Foster families may be the center of the team in this model. Foster families reach out to members of the birth family who are legally available and wish to participate. Other team members might be significant adults or, with older teens, close peers. Family advocates specially trained to facilitate the process and to empower parents are key to this model. The CFT identifies strengths and needs and seeks to address the needs both with formal treatment programs and with more natural supports such as jobs, sports programs, or other peer-based programs in the community. Getting caseworkers on board with this approach may be difficult, because it is radically different from what most have experienced. An evaluation program contracted by a community mental health system is producing promising data regarding outcomes when fidelity to a wraparound process is observed.

TFC programs or a wraparound process requires support of a special program. Training mental health care providers for work in such programs is important for improving services to youths in foster care; including more senior clinicians in such programs is essential for quality care. Senior clinicians must undo perceptions of elitism and arrogance and find ways of bonding with foster parents, who offer down-to-earth wisdom. Both need each other. Some clinicians are not able to work in this context. Psychiatrists (having been trained primarily in a biomedical model) who are too narrowly focused on providing medication services might be able to play a narrow role with the team but are not able to take a clinical leadership role. Community psychiatrists and mental health care providers who have similar skills relevant to work with specialized treatment programs for foster care children and who understand social contextual issues are more likely to be relevant to such programs. As in all innovative programs that break the mold, senior clinicians with standing in the community must stand as advocates with program administrators if such programs are to be supported by legislatures or private foundations.

■ CONCLUSIONS

Foster care programs offer insight into working in or consulting to the public welfare system. This chapter provides a description of how the public-sector system has evolved to provide protection and services to children with special requirements. Foster care children and their biological and foster care families need considerable attention and support. As the system develops with innovative programming, the level of care is expected to become more focused on the individual needs of the children and their families. Understanding what can be done to see this process through to fruition is the first step toward an attainable and realistic goal of child- and family-centered services.

■ REFERENCES

Adoption and Safe Families Act of 1997, Pub. L. No. 105-89

Adoption Assistance and Child Welfare Act of 1980, Pub. L. No. 96-272

Barth RP, Berry M: Implications of research on the welfare of children under permanency planning, in Child Welfare Research Review, Vol 1. Edited by Barth RP, Berrick JD, Gilbert N. New York, Columbia University Press, 1994, pp 323–368

Carmichael-Olson H, Morse BA, Huffine CW: Development and psychopathology: fetal alcohol syndrome and related conditions. Semin Clin Neuropsychiatry 3:262–284, 1998

Fine P: A Developmental Network Approach to Therapeutic Foster Care. Washington, DC, Child Welfare League of America, 1993

Gallagher MM, Leavitt KS, Kimmel HP: Mental health treatment of cumulatively/repetitively traumatized children. Smith College Studies in Social Work 65:205–237, 1995

Kates WG, Johnson RL, Rader MW, et al: Whose child is this? assessment and treatment of children in foster care. Am J Orthopsychiatry 61:584–591, 1991

Knitzer J: Unclaimed Children: The Failure of Public Responsibility to Children and Adolescents in Need of Mental Health Services. Washington, DC, Children's Defense Fund, 1982

Multiethnic Placement Act of 1994, Pub. L. No. 103-382, sec. 553

Pilowsky DJ: Short-term psychotherapy with children in foster care, in Psychotherapies With Children: Adapting the Psychodynamic Process. Edited by O'Brien JD, Pilowsky DJ, Lewis OW. Washington, DC, American Psychiatric Press, 1992, pp 291–311

Pumariega AJ, Winters NC (eds): The Handbook of Child and Adolescent Systems of Care: The New Community Psychiatry. San Francisco, CA, Jossey-Bass, 2003

Rosenfeld AA, Wasserman S: Healing the Heart: A Therapeutic Approach to Disturbed Children in Group Care. Washington, DC, Child Welfare League of America, 1990

Rosenfeld AA, Wasserman S, Pilowsky DJ: Psychiatry and children in the child welfare system. Child Adolesc Psychiatr Clin N Am 7:515–536, 1998

Steinhauser PD: The Least Detrimental Alternative: A Systematic Guide to Case Planning and Decision Making for Children in Care. Toronto, ON, University of Toronto Press, 1991

13 CONSULTATION TO CHILD CARE SETTINGS

Charles Keith, M.D.

Alice Long, M.A.

Since the late 1970s, full-time child care for preschool children has become increasingly common. Nationwide, approximately 50% of all preschool children are placed in organized, freestanding child care centers or in home-based child care (although in some communities such as Durham, North Carolina, where we are located, this figure approaches 65%–70%). Current economic, political, and philosophical trends will continue to push the majority of parents in the country to place their young children in child care for the foreseeable future. Therefore, bringing mental health services such as consultation to child care settings is a pressing yet often neglected issue (Bredekemp 1996; Eth et al. 1985; Furman 1995; Greenspan et al. 1975; Weiss and LaRoche 1989; Wesley 1994). The vast majority of child care programs in the country are financial shoestring operations, eking out an existence through minimum wages for staff and other fiscal strangulations. Interestingly, to our knowledge only one early child care system (i.e., tax-supported Head Start) requires that each of its programs have regular mental health consultation (Core 1970; Farley 1971; Hawks 1978; Mowder et al. 1993). As of 2003, the state of North Carolina had no requirements or guidelines for mental health consultation in child care settings. We assume that many if not most other states also lack this requirement.

Studies conducted over the past two decades have almost unanimously reached the conclusion that poorly run, understaffed child care settings are deleterious to child development. The consultation model we present in this chapter has the potential for helping to raise the quality of the entire child care program by improving teacher morale as well as bringing help to specific children. The model was developed and implemented by A. Long (one of the authors of this chapter) beginning in the mid-1970s in Durham, North Carolina, as an integral part of her role as director of the preschool program in the Division of Child and Adolescent Psychiatry at Duke University Medical Center.

In addition to the general principles of consultation, the child care consultant must be knowledgeable in the following areas:

- Early child development and its pathological variations
- The roles and limitations of parents in fostering or limiting normal development. Parents are not the responsible and sole agents for a child's development. Keeping this firmly in mind helps the consultant and the child care staff to be ever watchful for their tendency to blame the parent. Such blaming, if left unchecked, will only disrupt and destroy any hope for building a parental alliance. The younger the child, the greater the tendency to overidentify with the child and blame the parent.

On these issues, *Zero to Three,* the bulletin of the National Center for Clinical Infant Programs (http://www.zerotothree.org), will be of assistance to early childhood educators and consultants.

For clarity, we break down our consultation model into seven successive steps and describe the successes and pitfalls of each. We believe that our model has particular strengths around alliance building with teachers and parents, which is an absolute necessity if the consultant wishes to remain in the child care community over time. The seven steps are as follows:

1. Entry into the child care system
2. Entry into a specific child care center to consult concerning a child
3. Entry into a child care classroom to observe a specific child
4. Observation of the child
5. Consultant's interactions with the child care staff after observation of the child
6. Meeting with parents after the child observation and meeting with the classroom teacher
7. Handling the situation when the child care teacher is the problem

■ THE CONSULTATIVE PROCESS

Entry Into the Child Care System

The prospective consultant has the choice of whether to enter the child care system via a single child care setting and then expand to others, or to begin through contacts with an overarching child care organization. In the 1970s in Durham, a community-wide child care organization had just conducted a survey of child care directors that was sponsored by the League of Women Voters. Unsurprisingly, this survey indicated that large numbers of young children had emotional problems and needed mental health services. Armed with these survey results, our consultant decided to make a presentation before the community-wide child care organization to introduce herself and describe how she could help teachers and child care directors understand and work with problem children. The consultant's salary was paid by community mental health center funds, and hence she did not have to approach the child care directors or parents for funding. (We tried direct billing of parents and attempted to use Medicaid and insurance funding sources, all of which required an extensive registration process. This obstacle proved insurmountable, because consultation involved initial contacts with frightened, defensive parents who were only put off by immediate requests to register in the mental health system.)

In her initial presentation to the child care directors, the consultant emphasized her education and work background as a teacher who had struggled with and who understood the issues facing child care teachers, particularly how to work with a single child in the context of a group. It was our impression that those from other professional disciplines, such as psychology and psychiatry, might have to spend more effort and time to convince child care personnel that they understood these issues.

The consultant described her model of consultation (the same one outlined in this chapter) in some detail and emphasized that there would be no initial charge for her services. She announced that she would be calling the child care directors to set up an initial exploratory visit or consultation about specific children, and she stated that if a child care director did not wish to meet with her at that time, she would be available in the future.

Entry Into a Specific Child Care Center to Consult Concerning a Child

The consultant should insist on having an initial meeting with the director to establish a working alliance and to set the director's mind at ease as much as possible concerning the consultant's entry into the child care center. It is well known that agency personnel tend to be concerned about the potential for receiving criticism from consultants coming into their center; therefore, they erect barriers and defenses to ward off such a threat. This issue must be sufficiently worked through before the consultant can meet with a teacher and eventually observe and consult about a specific child.

Frequently, a child care director will ask the consultant for help with a child without first contacting the child's parent. The child care personnel may have had previous conflictive interactions with the parent of a problem child and might understandably wish not to repeat such exchanges. In such cases, the consultant should reiterate the very firm position that she cannot observe or consult concerning a specific child without having an agreement (and ideally an alliance) with the parent. The consultant should remind the child care personnel that any attempts to set up an intervention concerning a child will most likely fail unless the parent supports such an endeavor.

At this point, the child care director will often ask the consultant to make the initial contact with the parent to explain the situation. The consultant should respond that initial contact is the role of the child care director but that the consultant will help the director understand any issues involving the parent. The consultant could engage in role play with the director about how a telephone conversation or initial meeting might go with a frightened, defensive parent. In any initial meetings with the parent, the consultant may offer to sit with the director and can even take a leading role in such meetings, as long as the child care director is also present to emphasize that the child care center and the consultant are united in their efforts to help the parent and the child. If the parent refuses the consultation, the consultant will not observe the child but instead will consult with the director about general issues of handling children with such problems.

Entry Into a Child Care Classroom to Observe a Specific Child

Once the parent gives approval for the consultant to observe his or her child, the child care director will set up an appointment with the parent to discuss the observational findings. The appointment with the parent should take place before the classroom observation by the consultant. This establishes a time frame for the consultative process. The director should then approach the classroom teacher to clarify details of the consultation and how the consultant will observe the child. Before the actual observation of the child, the consultant should ask the teacher to briefly note simple observations of the child's behavior, verbalizations, and interactions with the staff and with other children. The teacher should be asked not to make any judgments or conclusions about the child but only to note specific behaviors. At a prearranged time, the consultant then enters the classroom, sitting in a chair at the side of the children's group, but neither in front nor in back if possible. The consultant should try to sit in a smaller chair so as not to tower over the group. The typical observation phase of the consultation requires 2–3 hours, during which time the consultant jots down specific observations similar to those he or she asked the teacher to make. Most teachers are initially nervous about the consultant observing their interactions with children, but after 2–3 hours the demands of the children and the inevitable group processes within the classroom help the teacher settle into his or her routine and not worry about the consultant's presence.

In addition, a lengthy observation gives the consultant an opportunity to observe the child in many activities, both structured and unstructured. Because most states require all children to go outside for recreational activities unless there is inclement weather, it is often possible to observe children outdoors in more open, free activities in contrast to the structured activities within a classroom. Morning observations are best, because both teachers and children are more refreshed, in contrast to the inevitable fatigue of the afternoon hours.

The teacher introduces the consultant as another teacher who has come to "watch children work and play." The parent may have told the particular child under observation that the consultant would be entering the classroom. However, the consultant should ask the teacher not to tell the child that he or she is the one specifically being watched. Considerable truth rests in the statement that the consultant is there to watch and learn how the children work and play in the classroom. In our years of experience, not telling a particular child that the consultant is there to watch him or her relieves some of the "spotlight" pressures of the consultation. At times, it is best not to be brutally honest.

Observation of the Child

Once comfortably seated, the consultant can then begin to observe and listen to the child and the milieu. It is always surprising how much can be learned by simply observing. The list of observable features and issues is lengthy, and only a few salient ones need be noted here:

1. What are the consultant's immediate impressions of the child? Note the child's clothing, cleanliness, and general appearance sui generis and in relation to the group.

2. What is the nature of the child's interactions with the group? Is there a balance between solitary and group interactional play? Do the group dynamics allow the child to engage in solitary play?

3. Is the child able to pay attention when the teacher provides structured instructional activities? What is the nature of the child's behavioral controls? Can the child contain his or her aggressive impulses, or does he or she frequently engage in shoving and pushing or touching other children or objects?

4. What is the child's affective and emotional expressional range? Is there continual agitation and tension or persistent sadness? Does the child appear fatigued or withdrawn? Does the child have a range of affects, from quiet pensiveness to excited interactions with others? Does the child fre-

quently appear angry, or is he or she angry only when intruded on by others? Does the child appear anxious and jittery, or can he or she be in a relaxed, calm state? Does the child always need to be in the spotlight, jostling and shoving his or her way into the teacher's favor, or can he or she share favors from the teacher with others?

5. What are the child's language capabilities? How can an observer assess language when not talking directly with the child? Although the observer may not be able to hear the content of interactional speech, note where and how the child interacts verbally with others and whether others respond in what appear to be appropriate verbal interactions. Is there an interest in language as created by the teacher and others, or does the observed child appear bored and unresponsive to verbal interactions?

6. Can the child engage in tasks and bring them to some kind of completion, or does he or she exhibit random, hyperactive motoric activity that disrupts attempts to focus on an intellectual task?

7. How does the child relate with authority figures, namely the teacher and his or her assistant? Is there active avoidance, or are there persistent struggles accompanied by defiance of group rules? Is there a wish to seek appropriate praise and pleasurable interactions with the teacher, or does the child seem uninterested in the teacher's responses?

It is crucial that the observer place these specific observations of the child within the context of the milieu. Problematic observations make sense only when they stand out or are different from the behaviors of the group as a whole. If the entire classroom group is hyperactive, distracted, or distressed, the observer should immediately suspect milieu problems, such as faulty teacher supports or teacher interactions with the group. Perhaps the group itself is composed of too many difficult, disturbed children with problematic behaviors and anxieties that reverberate through the entire group, including the staff. Perhaps the teaching staff is involved in stressful, conflictive behavior with the child care administration, which then spills out onto the children under their care.

The consultant takes brief notes from these multiple observations, which can later be expanded into a narrative form. The consultant will initially be an object of curiosity to the children in the classroom. The consultant should eschew interaction with the children as much as possible. This can be accomplished by immediately and politely directing the children's attention back to the group and teacher. The consultant should usually say a few reassuring words to the teacher at the end of the observation. The consultant must continually acknowledge to himself or herself that despite reassurances, his or her presence is typically experienced by the teacher as a potential source of criticism. The consultant could say a few words about how well the group performed during the observation under the guidance of the teacher. Before meeting with the parent, the consultant must have a meeting with the teacher to hear the teacher's concerns about the child's behavior vis-à-vis the group and his or her teaching methods.

Consultant's Interactions With Child Care Staff After Observation of the Child

It is crucial that the consultant listen respectfully and thoughtfully to the teacher's concerns. This builds an alliance and gives the consultant further clues as to the teacher's perceptions of the child and what strengths and problems the teacher brings to the teaching situation. A typical response from teachers in these postobservational sessions is that "nothing works." If the child performed relatively well during the observation, the teacher may say that it was a surprisingly good day but that most days are very discouraging and all techniques the teacher tries are to no avail. This response of "nothing works" has been described in school consultation literature over the decades and presents a crucial challenge for the consultant. The consultant can experience this response as a challenge to his or her professional expertise, leading the consultant to think, "Anything I suggest will also not work."

The consultant may ask the teacher to go over specifically what he or she has tried. This question illustrates to the teacher that the consultant is not accepting at face value the notion that nothing works, and that through further mutual discussion and working together they can possibly come up with something that has a chance of working. In the course of this conversation, the consultant should also ask how interactions with the child's parents have gone, as a means of assessing the child care center's view of the parents and their capacity to be allies with the teachers. If after the initial interactions in the postobservational interview the teacher still feels that nothing works, the consultant can then say, "Let me go over my observations and see if anything in what I saw might give us some clues about something that might be helpful." Our consultant has repeatedly noticed that as she goes over her simple, concrete observations, the teacher often relaxes, because the consultant's observations most likely validate the teacher's own perceptions. The teacher then feels relieved when the consultant does not point out anything the teacher has done wrong.

At this point, the consultant and teacher may be able to talk about a specific behavioral issue. A common observation by teachers is that a particular child is "always hitting someone." The harried teacher often has the perception that the hitting arises out of the blue or perhaps comes from something going on at home. The consultant may be able to present observations about what leads up to a hitting episode. For instance, one child may hit another when the latter child attempts to join the first child's play with another child. If the consultant is able to flush out some of the antecedents of the disturbing behavior, there may be an opportunity to raise the question, "In light of this, how can we figure out how to help the child?" In this model of consultation, the consultant should be wary of offering an immediate solution. The teacher may have had other experts give pat answers or prescribe solutions that did not work. By offering solutions to a teacher, the consultant often unwittingly denigrates the teacher's capacities and may be experienced as belittling despite having good intentions in offering a possible answer for problem behaviors.

If the meeting with the teacher has gone well enough up to this point, the consultant might offer suggestions concerning how a teacher could talk with a child about problematic behavior such as hitting. More importantly, the teacher may come up with an intervention that perhaps the consultant has not thought of or may not consider particularly suitable. However, if the teacher has thought of it and views it as his or her own, then in fact it has a good chance of being effective because it flows out of the teacher's confidence.

Teachers in our community frequently become skeptical of behavioral charts, time-out chairs, and other commonly used tools. In our local Head Start program, involving more than 400 children, time-out chairs and behavioral charts have been abandoned under this model. Instead, teachers have gained confidence in using their own verbal and personal interactions with the children to help reduce the problematic behaviors. The emphasis in this consultation model on building an alliance with the teacher and utilizing whatever solutions he or she can develop appears to have increased teacher morale. This is evidenced, for instance, by the fact that teachers now attend teacher meetings almost 100% of the time. Before this consultation, attendance at meetings was poor, and those who did attend were often skeptical and felt discouraged about the children under their care.

Meeting With Parents After the Child Observation and Meeting With the Classroom Teacher

At this point in the consultative process, the consultant can meet with the parents alone, although the teacher may join if he or she wishes. In particular, the child care operator, the person of authority in the setting, is invited to attend the meeting at least for the initial few minutes. The consultant goes through essentially the same process with the parents that was done with the teacher; namely, asking the parents what they have noticed about the child in terms of what happens at the child care center or in other settings in the child's life. The consultant then shares with the parents the observations made by both the consultant and the teacher and the tentative plan that has been worked out to help the child. The consultant emphasizes that the plan is only tentative and that the parents' input is crucial for whatever is done. The large majority of parents are in agreement with whatever the child care center wishes to do. Again, the emphasis in the meeting with the parents is building an alliance in case further interventions are needed either within the child care center or through referral to other mental health services in the community. Our experience with this consultation model suggests that more than 90% of the children observed and worked with by teachers and parents do not require referral to an outside mental health agency.

Handling the Situation
When the Child Care Teacher Is the Problem

If a child care director asks our consultant to observe a problematic teacher, our consultant will insist that the teacher be made aware of the reason he or she is being observed. To implement notification of the teacher, the consultant asks the director to meet with the teacher to discuss the director's concerns and to tell the teacher that the consultant has been asked to observe him or her in the classroom. Incidentally, Head Start guidelines require that each classroom and teacher be observed by a mental health consultant two times yearly.

▮ CONCLUSIONS

The consultation model presented in this chapter depends heavily on building alliances with child care directors and teachers over time. We were fortunate that our consultant, Ms. Long, served in this capacity for more than 25 years in our community, so she had the advantage of a good reputation when entering a child care center. We question whether any consultation model (this one or those emphasizing behavioral programming) can be truly effective unless time is spent building respectful working alliances with child care directors and teachers.

The training for and practice of mental health consultation in child care centers are not emphasized (and in many instances are not even present) in most mental health training programs. As society recognizes the effects of early, out-of-home child care on young children, consultation will emerge as a crucial resource for bringing our rich knowledge of early child development into the caretaking system.

▮ REFERENCES

Bredekemp S (ed): Developmentally Appropriate Practice in Early Childhood Programs, Revised Edition. Washington, DC, National Association for the Education of Young Children, 1996

Core HM: Mental health consultation in a Head Start program. Hosp Community Psychiatry 21:183–185, 1970

Eth S, Silverstein S, Pynoos RS: Mental health consultation to a preschool following the murder of a mother and child. Hosp Community Psychiatry 36:73–76, 1985

Farley GK: Mental health consultation with a Head Start center. J Am Acad Child Psychiatry 10:555–571, 1971

Furman E (ed): Preschoolers: Questions and Answers: Psychoanalytic Consultations With Parents, Teachers and Caregivers. Madison, CT, International Universities Press, 1995

Greenspan SI, Nover RA, Brunt CH: Mental health consultation to early child care, in The Practice of Mental Health Consultation. Edited by Mannino FV, MacLennan BW, Shore MF. Adelphi, MD, National Institute of Mental Health, 1975, pp 105–130

Hawks D: The Mental Health Consultant for Head Start, 2nd Edition. College Park, University of Maryland College Center for Professional Development, 1978

Mowder BA, Unterspan D, Knuter L, et al: Psychological consultation and Head Start: data, issues, and implications. Journal of Early Intervention 17:1–7, 1993

Weiss J, LaRoche C: The role of child psychiatrists as consultants to day cares. Can J Psychiatry 34:589–593, 1989

Wesley PW: Providing on-site consultation to promote quality in integrated child care programs. Journal of Early Intervention 18:391–402, 1994

14 DAY TREATMENT CENTERS/PARTIAL HOSPITALIZATION SETTINGS

Laurel J. Kiser, Ph.D., M.B.A.

Jerry D. Heston, M.D.

Marilyn Paavola, L.C.S.W.

Partial hospitalization programs (PHPs) for children and adolescents provide an intensive therapeutic experience designed to meet the needs of acutely and severely disturbed young patients. The combination of a highly structured, therapeutically intensive treatment plan and setting along with maintenance of family and community ties allows for the significant impact achieved by this modality. This same combination produces significant challenges for the professional staff and consultants who work within a partial hospitalization setting.

Early PHPs for children and adolescents in the 1960s utilized three basic models: 1) community-based services or clinics, 2) psychoeducational groups, or 3) developmental programs. Many programs were designed around the school year, with youngsters remaining in treatment for 1–3 years. Program funding included state and local support, health insurance, private payment, and education funds.

Despite its long history, the modality has been severely underutilized (Parker and Knoll 1990). Factors contributing to low utilization of PHPs included lack of definition, criteria, and outcome data; inadequate funding and insurance benefit limitations; and clinical issues related to clinician inexperience with the model and lack of resolve in the family for keeping a difficult child at home.

Recent industry trends (e.g., cost containment, managed care, prospective and negotiated payment plans) create more favorable conditions for partial hospitalization providers. Shifting practice patterns include substantial growth in the number of PHPs, increased utilization of acute partial hospitalization care for patient stabilization, and rapid development of a variety of intensive outpatient treatment options. An extensive discussion of ambulatory behavioral health service models is provided elsewhere (Kiser et al. 2002).

▮ DAY TREATMENT OR PARTIAL HOSPITALIZATION PRACTICE

Day treatment and *partial hospitalization* are umbrella terms describing hospital diversion care. With changes in behavioral health care delivery, a range of less costly and less restrictive treatment modalities fills gaps along the continuum of psychiatric care between inpatient and outpatient office visits. To provide definition and structure to these treatment alternatives, three levels of ambulatory behavioral health services have been outlined (Kiser et al. 1993, 1999). Partial hospitalization is the prototype for Level 1; this level also includes other intensive hospital diversion services providing crisis stabilization and acute symptom reduction. Level 2 services such as day treatment, after-school programs, or intensive outpatient programs (IOPs) provide stabilization, symptom reduction, and skills development. Level 3 represents the least intensive ambulatory level of services, providing coordinated treatment for relapse prevention. Certain characteristics differentiate these services from outpatient treatment: hours of weekly involvement; a coordinated, multimodal approach; and the ability to gain access to specified crisis intervention services. These services represent specific, more intensive levels of care than outpatient services, without the iatrogenic effects of hospitalization. Like inpatient services, PHPs and IOPs are intended to provide intensive, highly structured treatment. They do so by offering a menu of therapeutic interventions—individual, group, and family therapy; educational or vocational therapy; recreation and activity therapy; and medical and nursing services—tailored to the individual needs of the child or adolescent. This multimodal treatment is typically designed and delivered by a multidisciplinary team of professionals representing psychiatry, psychology, social work, educational or vocational therapy, occupational or recreational therapy, and nursing.

Regardless of the specific level of care examined, all ambulatory programs incorporate two basic philosophies into their mission: 1) they strive to treat patients with intensive treatment needs while limiting the disruption caused to the patients' normal daily routine, and 2) the providers must therefore clearly delineate their admission and discharge criteria to reflect who can be safely and effectively treated within their treatment setting.

In addition, partial hospitalization or ambulatory programs take advantage of family and community supports and strengths in designing treatment. From the perspective of providers of services to children and adolescents, this treatment design translates "into a program of therapeutic interventions designed to maintain power within the parental/familial subsystem and to view that subsystem as competent in providing care for the child" (Heston et al. 1996, p. 878). These core values are seen at various levels within an ambulatory treatment program despite variations in orientation, intensity, or location.

Partial hospitalization and other ambulatory behavioral health services take place in organizational settings such as multiservice mental health organizations; general, pediatric, or psychiatric hospitals; and freestanding facilities (Culhane et al. 1994). Locations for partial hospitalization services can be varied. Siting partial hospitalization services away from hospital facilities has the advantage of diluting the possible stigma associated with psychiatric inpatient care and in some cases decreases overhead cost. Schools, community centers, and outpatient clinics—settings closely connected with the everyday activities of children and adolescents—are logical sites for child and adolescent ambulatory behavioral health services.

Organizational Models

Partial hospitalization and other ambulatory behavioral health services are structured in various ways. Both closed and open staffing models (discussed in "Communication" later in this chapter) can be implemented effectively within the context of a well-functioning multidisciplinary team. Hierarchical models for ambulatory care also range from highly structured vertical systems to more egalitarian approaches. From a systems theory perspective, it seems logical that a healthy and functional staff will provide the most effective care. Programs that promote direct, open communication; clear role definition and boundaries; effective leadership that empowers staff members; and job satisfaction provide an organizational structure that will support healthy team functioning.

The composition, organization, and functioning of this team can differ significantly from one program to another. Some examples are listed below:

- *A psychoeducational program designed around a classroom model.* Teachers and teachers' aides are the primary staff members involved with daily patient care. Therapists may interact with students only during scheduled therapy sessions, which may take place either during or after program hours.

• *A hospital-based unit designed around an inpatient model.* The primary staff members involved with daily patient care are usually nurses and psychiatric technicians. Social workers or counselors lead daily groups, multifamily groups, and the like. Consulting or contracting professionals (psychiatrists, psychologists, nurses, and social workers) provide individual and family therapy outside the program milieu.

• *A general psychiatry unit designed around a systems theory model.* Staff members with primary responsibilities for daily patient care are teachers, activity therapists, recreational therapists, nurses, and other related staff. Clinical staff members (psychiatrists, psychologists, nurses, and social workers) provide individual, group, and family psychotherapy to the patients as part of the multidisciplinary team.

Practicing in a Partial Hospitalization Setting

Although each staff member may have a different function on the team, all work together to provide a unified therapeutic environment for each patient. The descriptions of roles and responsibilities for staff positions provided below illustrate how the different positions interact and interrelate and define boundaries where they clearly exist.

Leadership roles in PHPs and ambulatory behavioral health services are critical to the success of a therapeutic program. Child and adolescent services require an on-site director who has the education and clinical experience specific to the needs of the target patient population (Block et al. 1991) and who is also a treatment team member actively involved in managing the therapeutic environment.

In PHPs that provide acute symptom reduction and crisis intervention services as an alternative to hospitalization, a medical director—ideally a board eligible or board certified child and adolescent psychiatrist—who is medically and clinically responsible for the program's patients is an essential member of the treatment team. The medical director leads the treatment team and coordinates a patient's treatment in conjunction with the other team professionals. The psychiatrist's role within ambulatory services that provide less intensive care depends on the specific philosophy of the organization, but programs should minimally provide medical or psychiatric consultation for patients as needed (Kiser et al. 1993).

Psychologists, social workers, nurses, and mental health counselors on staff serve at various times in multiple roles, providing different forms of therapy (individual, family, and group). These clinicians also provide specialized services such as conducting psychological testing of individual patients and family members as needed, developing specialized behavioral plans, and taking social histories. Social workers also serve as consultants to the treatment team on social services issues and community resources. Within ambulatory behavioral health services, in which team functioning is critical to providing therapeutic services, we recommend that clinicians develop a sense of team identity, best accomplished when 1) a proportion (at least 60%) of their time is spent providing care within a specific service, 2) they carry a consistent case load, and 3) they regularly participate in multidisciplinary team meetings and programmatic staff development activities.

Many PHPs incorporate case managers, who are assigned to provide overall direction to a patient's therapeutic program. The case manager has primary responsibility for planning and coordinating the patient's treatment within the program (and perhaps at other levels of care within the system) by 1) developing a treatment plan identifying the patient's psychological and emotional strengths and weaknesses, 2) outlining needed therapy contracts, 3) establishing appropriate discharge goals, 4) conducting liaison with outside agencies, and 5) maintaining continuity of care as the patient makes transitions to more or less intensive levels of care.

If there is a nurse on the team, he or she assists the staff by conducting an initial nursing assessment; dispensing medications and monitoring the effects on patients; and charting patients' height, weight, and vital signs. The nurse can provide group instruction on health-related topics. Direct-care patient services are often supervised by a charge nurse, nurse manager, floor coordinator, or other nursing staff member. This individual's primary responsibility is to maintain adequate and appropriate coverage (supervision) of patients during program hours by developing the daily or weekly schedule and also coordinating coverage for staff absences and vacation time. In all the models listed in "Organizational Models" above, the direct-care staff provides specialized services needed to maintain the therapeutic milieu, including education, recreation activities, social skills exercises, and community meetings. These team members provide frontline patient coverage and are primarily responsible for maintaining the behavior management program.

Finally, a support staff (e.g., secretaries, administrative assistants, office managers) is key to successful program operation. These individuals provide a foundation for program activities by taking initial intake information, organizing the office, and providing general reception and secretarial functions for the program.

The treatment team itself is the core of best practices for the partial hospitalization setting. Therefore, it is crucial for PHPs and other ambulatory behavioral health services to provide a variety of mechanisms to manage the complexities common to this kind of integrated system, such as those described in the sections that follow.

Staff Empowerment

The multidisciplinary team must operate from a philosophy that every individual team member provides a unique perspective to treatment and that each person's opinion is valued and incorporated into the program of therapeutic activities. Valuing and empowering all staff members enhances team members' commitment and investment in therapeutic interventions, thereby contributing to the effectiveness of treatment.

This basic philosophy begins with the administration and those in leadership roles. The philosophy may be implemented in various ways. One way is to develop a distinctive job description for each team member and, through a collaborative effort between the team member and the supervisor, incorporate the talents and strengths of that member for the team's benefit. Efforts to include each member in the organization's overall performance improvement plan can help promote a philosophy of total team commitment and can considerably improve practice in general. Regular (annual or semiannual) job evaluations and job satisfaction surveys provide further opportunities to maintain this philosophy, because each member reflects on ways to enhance his or her own performance and provides valuable input regarding problem areas. Participation by all staff members in ongoing program development allows each team member to have a voice and an active sense of program ownership.

Communication

The efficacy of partial hospitalization and ambulatory behavioral health services depends to a great extent on good communication. When a group of well-trained professionals works as a team, a clear power hierarchy is established. A multitiered system is one effective approach; it may include the administrative/clinical management tier (responsible for program operations, personnel, and finances), the program coordinator (responsible for professional services and program schedules), and the direct-care tier (responsible for patient coverage). The decision-making style adopted by this group and also the channels it uses for communicating information and decisions set the overall tone for all staff-level interactions. Communication can be formal (e.g., regularly scheduled clinical staff meetings, treatment planning team meetings, clinical case consultations, direct-care staff meetings, administration meetings, staff development activities, and individual supervision). These organized communications provide critical structure to the exchange of information. In fact, scheduling daily meetings to address treatment concerns is recommended in the *Standards and Guidelines for Child and Adolescent Partial Hospitalization* (Block et al. 1991).

Effective communication in informal settings, such as day-to-day exchanges among team members, is an important means of sharing clinical information and opportunities to give support. It is important to provide time, availability, and leadership for informal communication. Encouraging the staff to share lunch times or to meet for social or recreational activities can allow for such opportunities of informal communication. Informal gatherings after treatment hours to allow everyone to decompress are also beneficial. Helping staff members to set appropriate boundaries between work and personal relationships is a necessary precaution regarding informal communication and support. The following example illustrates how both formal and informal communication approaches were used:

> When the director of a PHP became aware of several splits (both theoretical and personal) in the clinical staff, she led a series of group supervision staff meetings. In conjunction with this effort, the staff was encouraged to do charting in the staff office rather than in private offices. A potluck luncheon was scheduled, and the staff participated in several after-work social events (happy hours), which resulted in a more cohesive staff. This combination of formal and informal communication resulted in a much more functional treatment team.

In closed staff models in which the entire treatment team, including admitting physicians, operates consistently with relatively little influence from outside professionals, informal communication may occur more easily because of the availability and predictability of team members. This contributes to a highly therapeutic milieu. Conversely, in open staff models in which staff members rotate in and out and different attending physicians with varying management styles lead treatment, formal communication is more frequently used to address team and patient issues, and delays in implementation may occur because of the unavailability of key staff members at critical moments. All in all, effective and frequent communication cannot be overemphasized for healthy team functioning.

Supervision

Two types of supervision can be provided: *group supervision* and *individual supervision*. Each team member can participate in group supervision experiences (e.g., clinical care meetings, direct care meetings, group process meetings). Individual supervision and consultation may involve each staff member assigned to a specific supervisor; the amount of supervision provided depends on the discipline and on the training level, experience, and performance appraisal of the staff member. Regardless of the independent practice status of staff members, supervision and consultation can provide avenues for sharing clinical information, problem solving on difficult cases, and promoting professional support and guidance.

Flexibility

Flexibility is a key component of successful practice. When the patient population treated by a PHP is more severely ill, the treatment team faces increased challenges for maintaining a therapeutic program:

> A successful partial hospitalization program began receiving heavy referrals of patients with serious emotional disturbance and severe acting-out behaviors. Admissions were scheduled to be as dispersed as possible to maintain the existing therapeutic milieu. However, the team experienced increasing challenges due to short lengths of stay and increased problem severity.

The team can respond in several ways: 1) it can incorporate new patients into the already existing milieu, expecting that time will be needed to shape new behaviors but risking negative effects to the milieu; 2) program leaders can watch for contagion and guard against the team reacting or tending to "put out fires" by separating the more severely acting-out patients—and maintaining a functional group of patients with necessary but minimal staff coverage; or 3) the team can be creative and flexible, with smaller treatment teams of direct-care and clinical team members who develop and treat smaller, manageable communities in a self-contained area.

These are but a few responses that a well-developed team may incorporate in a difficult and challenging milieu. Flexibility in treatment methods is also a necessary part of practice within a PHP. For example, given the type of children and adolescents presenting for care and the function of PHPs, traditional one-on-one individual therapy may not be as effective as clinicians being present in the classroom or during recreational activities to assist patients in coping with difficult situations or applying newly acquired anger management skills. This intervention method allows patients to respond to situations in a realistic manner and hopefully will ensure their success after discharge. Clinicians may also encourage family participation in the milieu by inviting parents to attend daily activities so they can observe interventions and can support or confront their child as needed. Group therapies may require adjustment to fit the milieu and the population being treated (e.g., the needs of children and adolescents in PHPs might be better met by more task-oriented groups or interactive playgroups designed to enhance the patient's ability to interact with others than by insight-oriented process groups). In short, when serving a more challenging patient population, being a creative and flexible clinician increases the likelihood of a successful treatment program.

Networking

In partial hospitalization settings, it is important to maintain an extensive network of referrals and community-based professional and agency contacts. If the focus is to treat severely disturbed children and adolescents in a short period of time, then it is imperative that an extensive support network be established. Such a network permits transferring patients to other levels of care smoothly and successfully. The network may include the school system, other mental health professionals, the juvenile justice system, children's services, in-home services, and so forth. Successful clinicians—those who focus on effective dispositions from the admission day—may be seen inviting representatives of these various agencies to the intake session or to the initial family therapy session (with family consent) to make the greatest use of resources for the family.

█ CONSULTATION TO PARTIAL HOSPITALIZATION AND DAY TREATMENT PROGRAMS

Having described different models and the general practice of partial hospitalization, we now focus on consultations to PHPs. Consultations may be directed toward a specific patient or client issue; they may be focused on a particular aspect of the program or individual requesting the consultation; or they may be directed to an entire system, such as when a program changes its practice model in response to new problems in its population or changes in funding sources (Caplan 1970).

Consultants are frequently asked for an opinion about some aspect of a patient's care. Such clinical case consultations to a psychiatrist may be about medications, to a clinical psychologist about developing a behavioral plan, or to an experienced family therapist about seeking a second opinion regarding an impasse in therapy. Common to each of these examples, as well as to more systemic consultations, is an assessment that involves gathering information, organizing it, and disseminating it to the consultee, the PHP. Pitfalls can occur at each step in the process.

Gathering Information

Although getting information from multiple sources is a standard concept for most clinicians, it cannot be underestimated in assessments of patients in a PHP. This guideline may especially apply to outpatient practitioners, who tend to rely heavily on patient and family reports because they are most readily available outside a structured program. Direct interviews with patients and parents are valuable, but the multidisciplinary staff of a PHP has a wealth of information that may be used. This information includes ratings, categorizations, observations, opinions, views, and deductions.

The information may be mined in several ways. Traditional psychiatric or psychological therapy usually follows a model that begins with a direct evaluation before obtaining information from teachers and others involved with a patient. The risk of using this model when consulting is that the refer-ral source (the PHP) may perceive that the consultant values the information obtained from the patient over that obtained from the consultee. This percep-tion should be avoided. Gathering information from the program staff can be done differently depending on the PHP model with which one is working. Scheduled staff meetings are frequently the major setting in which informa-tion is passed. Successful consultants listen carefully to all team members and encourage participation by the entire staff. Some consultants also have or cre-ate opportunities to communicate with various staff members outside formal staff meetings. Collecting this information helps the consultant function more effectively.

Regardless of the method chosen to obtain information, the consultant must approach PHP team members as professionals in their field. Allowing staff members to talk about patients in their own terms is helpful. Misunder-standings can occur if the clinician assumes he or she knows what the teacher or other staff members mean when they use language that is not the primary clinical vernacular of the consultant (e.g., when PHP teachers report that a client "is not SED"–i.e., does not have a serious emotional disturbance) but the consulting psychiatrist has diagnosed major depressive disorder. Consul-tants should understand the terms a teacher uses, as well as the vocabulary of allied therapists (e.g., art therapists and recreational therapists) who may work in PHPs. Consultants are encouraged to ask about unfamiliar concepts. Much is gained through this kind of respectful exchange.

Recognizing Differences Between Staff Views

In gathering information from various sources, consultants must beware of different perspectives between various staff members. Such differences may involve any team member and can occur at any point in the course of a pa-tient's admission to a PHP, from initial evaluation (including conflicts over the appropriateness of admission), through treatment planning, to transition and discharge. Discordant views regarding a particular patient may reflect ac-tual complexities in the case with which the staff is struggling. On the other hand, differing views may suggest team-related miscommunications that can negatively affect the patient's treatment.

Patient–Staff Conflicts

During the course of a patient-oriented consultation or during longitudinal follow-up of a patient's progress, a patient may report conflicts with specific staff members. The consultant must look for ways to share this information with the treatment team in a manner complementary to the patient's overall treatment. Consultants therefore must be aware of patient issues that may increase such reporting (e.g., patients with borderline personality disorder who engage in splitting behavior, patients with conduct disorders attempting to avoid responsibility). Consultants must also know the dynamics of the staff with which they are working (e.g., a certain activity therapist may have a confrontational style that may need modifying when dealing with anxious or unusually fragile patients). The consultant brings patient and staff issues together to improve the overall treatment.

Milieu Dysfunction

Besides individual patient variables and the interactions between staff members, the consultant must also be cognizant of the following:

- Milieu problems may affect a patient's treatment plan. Milieus that are unstable may amplify psychopathology.
- Patients who do not improve as expected or who worsen during the PHP admission must have their cases reviewed to determine the influence of negative milieu factors. Such influences may come from other patients and their families, the outside community, the staff, the physical space, or the program schedule.

The consultant must examine these issues and bring them into the final analysis and presentation to the treatment team.

Consultant–Staff Disagreement

During the course of consultation on a specific patient, divergent views between the treatment team and the consultant may emerge. To minimize this possible roadblock, the consultant must carefully identify the reason for the consultation. Rather than being asked simply to provide diagnosis, treatment, or some other specific service to a particular patient, PHP consultants are also called on to help the staff provide the most effective treatment to the patient or program component in question. Although disagreements can degenerate into arguments about what is best for a patient, consultants must avoid this pitfall and help the treatment team improve patient care. Rather than seeing the PHP or consultee as being noncompliant, the consultant must work to understand the reasons for the differences and use this information to improve the team's work with the patient. Because significant disagreements preclude effective consultation, the consultant must sometimes (although rarely) excuse himself or herself from the consultation. Bringing a new consultant with a different orientation into the process may help.

Advocating

Finally, as managed care grows and continues to influence psychiatric care, clinical consultants may be expected to help programs, patients, and their families negotiate appropriate financial coverage for treatment. Clinicians and physicians consulting with PHPs are frequently asked to review cases that have been tagged as questionable by the managed care company. The effective consultant needs to document the rationale for partial hospitalization treatment and should be familiar with medical necessity criteria and effective arguments for justifying appropriate treatment specific to the needs of each patient. Multiple opportunities exist within child and adolescent partial hospitalization and ambulatory behavioral health services for mental health consultation focused at the organizational level. Examples are detailed in the next section, "Staff Relations and Functions."

Staff Relations and Functions

Treating moderately to severely disturbed children and adolescents with acute symptoms and maintaining them within their home and community settings present both tremendous opportunities and challenges. Effective intervention in ambulatory settings requires a healthy and functional treatment team. Team problems (e.g., interpersonal dynamics, personality conflicts, power struggles, job dissatisfaction, and staff stress and burnout) quickly reverberate throughout the therapeutic milieu.

Consultants working with treatment teams can take various approaches:

- Active intervention with the team (e.g., group process sessions, direct confrontation of problems, discussions of roles and responsibilities) can be productive.
- Group work on team functioning provides an excellent opportunity for uncovering functional and dysfunctional formal and informal communication channels within the team. Offering great potential for success, these group sessions can be quite stressful and can cause significant discomfort for some staff members who are not accustomed to personal sharing in the work setting.
- Consultants must stay alert to the potential for increased problems within the PHP milieu while the consultative process is ongoing. The consultant and program administration must closely monitor this potential to ensure that problems within the team are not creating a caustic treatment environment.
- Finally, consultants must be aware that not all professionals are able to function successfully within ambulatory behavioral health care settings.

Some may require a greater sense of control over their moderately to severely disturbed patients or may be uncomfortable with the limited ability to directly affect the patient's home or community network. Discovering the person-to-environment fit necessary to function successfully in this setting is critical to helping teams and individuals conclude that staff changes may be the best response to some dysfunctional situations.

Keeping Current

Ambulatory behavioral health services is a rapidly developing field. Innovations in service design and delivery, clinical decision making, standards for care, and accountability occur with such rapidity that many ambulatory behavioral health services have difficulty keeping current. Program modifications include treatment adjustments to accommodate shorter lengths of stay, additions of tracks to target new patient groups, and modifications to medical records and information systems. Service-oriented journals and professional organizations such as the Association for Ambulatory Behavioral Healthcare provide information on benchmarking, current industry trends, standards and guidelines for partial hospitalization and other ambulatory programs, and networking with colleagues in the field. The publications and annual meetings of such organizations provide opportunities for continuing education.

Funding

Consultants should be familiar with the fiscal operations and challenges of ambulatory services. Several basic facts are important to remember:

- PHPs and other ambulatory behavioral health services operate at a significantly lower profit margin than inpatient units.
- Child and adolescent ambulatory services are more expensive to deliver than adult services.
- Relatively high and fixed staff costs are a necessary and large part of the ambulatory service budget.
- Seasonal census fluctuations are a normal part of ambulatory service delivery (especially with child and adolescent populations).
- Multiple sources of funding need to be explored, including indemnity insurance, managed care contracts under case rate or capitation models, and education dollars.

Integration of Services

Integrating PHPs or ambulatory behavioral health services within systems of care is becoming increasingly important. Development of a flexible continuum of services requires understanding different levels of care and expeditiously handling transitions between levels of care. Helping systems integrate ambulatory behavioral health services into an overall continuum requires a focus on access to and movement along the continuum, communication and information sharing between levels of care, and staff integration. However, directors of outpatient group practices or inpatient facilities often recognize the need for expanded services such as PHPs or IOPs but do not recognize the required special expertise to successfully provide quality care within ambulatory modalities. Consultants familiar with the provision of care within these levels provide valuable resources to the service system development team. Likewise, consultants to ambulatory treatment services can aid in developing admission and discharge criteria, transition policies and procedures, charting and documentation requirements, and other elements that meet the needs of the ambulatory team, diminish competition between levels of care, and are consistent with an integrated delivery system.

Because transition is a primary function of ambulatory care, staff members need to understand and appreciate the types of services delivered at both more intensive and less intensive levels of care. Preparing staff to meet the challenges of a true continuum is best accomplished by cross-training clinical staff members in programs at differing levels of intensity. Developing staff policies that allow clinical staff members to follow patients as they move between levels of care helps ensure continuity. However, continuity-of-care needs must be balanced with developing a core staff that maintains a sense of program identity.

▌ CONCLUSIONS

Clearly, PHPs and other ambulatory behavioral health services provide abundant professional opportunities for participation at a staff or consultative level. Modalities offering care along the continuum between traditional outpatient and inpatient treatment present a great deal of promise and many challenges. The dedication and commitment of team members and experts in partial hospitalization and ambulatory behavioral health services are continually tested in efforts to treat severely disturbed children and adolescents within settings that provide structure, supervision, and restrictiveness in the least amount possible while maintaining the safety and security of each patient. When such efforts are successful, the rewards are significant.

▌ REFERENCES

Block BM, Arney K, Campbell DJ, et al: Standards and Guidelines for Child and Adolescent Partial Hospitalization. Alexandria, VA, American Association for Partial Hospitalization, 1991

Caplan G: The Theory and Practice of Mental Health Consultation. New York, Basic Books, 1970

Culhane DP, Hadley TR, Kiser LJ: A national profile of partial hospital programs. Continuum 1:81–93, 1994

Heston JD, Kiser LJ, Pruitt DB: Child and adolescent partial hospitalization, in Child and Adolescent Psychiatry: A Comprehensive Textbook, 2nd Edition. Edited by Lewis M. Baltimore, MD, Williams & Wilkins, 1996, pp 883–890

Kiser LJ, Lefkovitz PM, Kennedy LL, et al: The continuum of ambulatory mental health services. Behav Healthc Tomorrow 2:14–16, 1993

Kiser LJ, King R, Lefkovitz PM: Comparison of practice patterns and a model continuum of ambulatory behavioral health services. Psychiatr Serv 50:605–618, 1999

Kiser LJ, Heston JD, Pruitt DB: Child and adolescent partial hospitalization and ambulatory behavioral health services, in Child and Adolescent Psychiatry: A Comprehensive Textbook, 3rd Edition. Edited by Lewis M. Philadelphia, PA, Lippincott Williams & Wilkins, 2002, pp 1083–1091

Parker S, Knoll JL 3rd: Partial hospitalization: an update. Am J Psychiatry 147:156–160, 1990

15 CHEMICAL DEPENDENCE PROGRAMS

Peter R. Cohen, M.D.

T he plot of the movie musical *West Side Story* reverberates with a drama similar to what the professional faces in consulting with chemical dependence programs. In this modernized version of *Romeo and Juliet,* two star-crossed lovers represent different sides of ethnic and turf conflicts between New York City gangs. If the musical were created today, alcohol, drugs, and other substances would be more central to the story. The star-crossed lovers in the clinical story would be the patient and his or her beloved substances of abuse that refuse to separate. Significant others will try to disrupt or maintain this unholy alliance. Arriving late on the scene, you are asked to evaluate and rescue some extremely difficult cases. You step into an arena of energy and chaos that begs to be resolved with better outcomes. Like the musical's gang members protecting their own interests, the major contending participants in the patient's life try to quell or threaten to disrupt the whole treatment process with their familiar refrains: 1) professionals who don't appreciate chemical dependence ("Hey, you've got a social disease!"); 2) Alcoholics Anonymous ("Don't get hot, 'cause man, you got some hard times ahead"; "Take it slow, and Daddy-O, you can live it up and die in bed!"); 3) families and peers who don't understand addiction but think they are helping by moralizing—and who ultimately support character pathology ("When you're a Jet, you stay a Jet!"); 4) families in desperation holding out against hope ("There's a place for us, somewhere a place for us"); 5) peers and gangs who promote defiance

("Here come the Jets, yeah, and we're gonna beat every last buggin' gang on the whole buggin' street"); and 6) managed care, which can help or restrict care ("Everything's free…for a small fee!…in America!").

This musical analogy sets the stage for general observations and advice to the community mental health practitioner and consultant. Substance abuse and dependence ultimately result in chaotic functioning on biological, psychological, and social levels. Mental health professionals' credibility as practitioners, consultants, and directors is dependent on being well versed—from a variety of perspectives—in the history and current knowledge of substance use and dependence.

This chapter describes the steps to approach practice and consultation for adolescent chemical dependence programs. It is hoped that these steps transform the inherent chaos of chemical dependence into improved somatic and mental health, safety for all concerned, self-sufficiency, and sustaining mutual reliance. For the sake of brevity, the terms *chemical* and *substance* are used interchangeably, as are *dependence* and *addiction*.

▮ STEPS FOR WORKING WITH ADOLESCENT CHEMICAL DEPENDENCE PROGRAMS

Step 1: Understand Teenage Chemical Dependence

Community mental health practitioners and consultants need to understand adolescent development and the issues concerning adolescent substance abuse in the context of treatment programs and the existing system of care. There is a special approach to these types of kids. A naïve or clueless practitioner will lose credibility or will simply be labeled a medicator or some other pejorative term by the program staff, the patients, and the patients' families.

The dynamics of the identity formation and biopsychosocial reorganization that occur during adolescence give special color and shade to substance abuse. Differentiating between typical goofy teenage behavior and a manifestation of addiction is critical. Abuse of alcohol and other drugs by teenagers is not simply a symptom of individuation or establishment of identity. Development becomes disrupted in youths with substance abuse problems. Their Global Assessment of Functioning (GAF) scores are plummeting. They are preoccupied with acquiring and abusing substances. They deny, minimize, or rationalize their chemical use and tend to have other complicating problems and diagnoses secondary to accompanying family, developmental, and social factors. Other family members and peers usually have a history of addictions and support the patient's continuing use.

A community mental health practitioner and consultant who is trained in certain psychotherapeutic modalities might be alarmed by the intense confrontation of a patient's behavior and past substance abuse by staff and patients in a chemical dependence and co-occurring disorder (COD) treatment program. However, direct confrontation can be very effective in treating a patient's minimization and denial. A community mental health practitioner and consultant must attend to how confrontation is delivered and help weigh the pros and cons of the message, the timing, and the follow-up.

Unfortunately, some community mental health practitioners and consultants who present themselves as chemical dependence specialists focus on the symptoms more than the syndrome and believe that reducing a particular symptom or anxiety will make patients less likely to abuse chemicals again. No research supports this approach. Regardless of overall health and GAF score, addicts will continue to use if they do not accept the disease and the need for social supports or a higher power in recovery.

Step 2: Understand the Difference Between Chemical Dependence Treatment and Therapy

Treatment requires that the patient master specific skills before beginning psychotherapy. In chemical dependence treatment, a patient needs to learn and consistently apply the following: Alcoholics Anonymous (AA)/Narcotics Anonymous (NA) steps; self-calming, stress management, and relapse prevention techniques; social skills; management of dysphoria; and ways to give and receive criticism constructively. Patients also need to receive continuing academic and substance education and to attend and actively comply with a treatment plan. Acquiring these skills permits a patient to explore past traumas and unresolved intrapsychic and family conflicts.

Appreciating the difference between treatment of addiction and psychotherapy helps avoid the usual conflicts between mental health treatment and chemical dependence treatment. Mental health therapy is based on the assumption that the patient has acquired or can learn higher-level skills in a progressive fashion. Addictive substances tend to cause fixation or regression of development, which cannot be repaired quickly. Establishing the building blocks of normal functioning and a commitment to receive help are major goals for an addicted teenager, which is why treatment cannot be ignored. As an example, an addicted girl who was raped is experiencing posttraumatic stress disorder. A premature focus on treating her trauma may result in further regression or relapse because she does not have the following skills to help her hold herself together: 1) calming skills, 2) acceptance of the need for help, 3) methods for staying sober, 4) awareness of how to stay away from further trouble, and 5) the ability to take responsibility for placing herself in precarious situations of drug and alcohol abuse in which a rapist would be more likely to appear (without relinquishing the ability to condemn the horror of being raped regardless of the circumstances).

A "model, but somewhat passive and depressed" teenager was about to graduate from a COD therapeutic day program. Near the end of his last school year, he was arrested for vandalism with another peer in the program and admitted that he had restarted using lysergic acid diethylamide (LSD). Some school staff members, having invested a lot of time and care in the patient, were enraged and wanted to expel him immediately and not let him graduate. Others on the staff wanted to interpret his regression as a response to recent family problems and feelings of loss and rejection by a parent (thereby therapizing the problem). The clinician treating the patient with interpersonal psychotherapy and antidepressant medication was asked to consult with the school about how to proceed with the patient. The clinician supported neither the punitive measures nor the "therapizing" recommended by staff. This patient had learned a great amount from treatment but was displaying a characteristic pattern of chemical dependence relapse. Needing to get back to the basics of NA/AA, he would regard the punitiveness as another rejection without understanding it and would interpret the therapizing as giving him permission to abuse LSD again without consequences. Psychic pain, if present, would surface in the treatment context. Treatment and limit setting were recommended instead. The school would expel him and not permit him to graduate until he fulfilled the following requirements, which paralleled the first five NA and AA steps: 1) having frequent reported contact with his sponsor and treatment group to reexamine the first step of NA/AA, 2) making a full confession of his behavior and receiving feedback from his peers, 3) making amends with his peers and program by coming up with an active plan by a certain date, 4) adhering to consequences at home and school concerning his responsibilities and whereabouts, and 5) having frequent and reported attendance at NA/AA. He complied with the plan and "sweated bullets" about how he would make amends with his peers and the program. On follow-up, he took full responsibility for coordinating and running the food concessions at the end-of-year school fair; he attended NA and AA faithfully to the point where he was leading groups; and he graduated from school and stayed committed to a sober program.

By understanding the difference between treatment and therapy, the community mental health practitioner and consultant can help a program staff define the vision and goals for its patients.

Step 3: Understand the Nature of the Treatment Program

The following list highlights the major lessons this clinician has learned as a consultant, treatment team member, and medical director at almost every level of care for chemical dependence and CODs:

1. Effective assessment and treatment require a program to identify with one or more components of a continuum of care. Clearly defined goals and an operational-structure program mission and vision are critical. Treatment Improvement Protocols distributed by the Center for Sub-

stance Abuse Treatment provide the essentials of adolescent substance abuse assessment and treatment (Winters 1999a, 1999b).

2. Program structures are relatively similar because they include the disciplines of chemical dependence counselors, therapists, and supervisors. As treatment intensity and clinical problem complexity increase, programs may include social workers, nurses, psychologists, expressive therapists, case managers, and psychiatric technicians. Inpatient programs also require psychiatrists and pediatricians as members of the treatment team, whereas outpatient programs may vary this role regarding diagnostic evaluations, medication therapy and monitoring, treatment team planning, and consultation. Regrettably, some outpatient programs ignore comorbidity in this population by viewing psychiatric diagnosis and treatment as a last resort for a resistant adolescent. Some crossover of roles between professional disciplines as well as respect of the traditional boundaries regarding tasks and expertise is expected. In any treatment program, frontline workers (usually the counselors, psychiatric technicians, and nurses) are those absorbing and managing the teenager's moment-to-moment primitive affects, thoughts, and behaviors. Social workers manage a balance between the needs of the family and those of the adolescent. Respect the thankless roles these professionals play by recognizing the energy and strength needed and by encouraging creativity, flexibility, and improvement in clinical expertise.

3. Components of treatment programs at different levels of care vary according to the intensity of the program and limitations on the length of stay. Common to all ideal programs are a) an evaluative component, b) drug and alcohol education, c) confrontational techniques, d) AA/NA 12-step orientation and meetings, e) group treatment modalities, f) multiple and individual family therapy, g) casework and case management, and h) an aftercare component. A therapeutic-community treatment perspective seems to be most effective in residential or intensive day programs. Sensitive to the lack of success in treating teenagers with disruptive disorders in a group setting, some programs favor individual and family approaches and use motivational techniques to move from a precontemplative to a contemplative stage of change and encourage sobriety. However, further research into understanding the effectiveness of program components and techniques in treating adolescents with different levels of substance use and psychopathology is needed.

4. Referrals to treatment come from a variety of sources. Consultants should be alert to the underlying motivations of a referral. A significant number of referrals usually come from the juvenile court system as a con-

dition of sentencing or as a deterrent to incarceration and allow some leverage to retain teenagers and their families in treatment. But judges and juvenile justice workers may become impatient with the deliberations of assessment or treatment programs. Referrals from families and schools can be accompanied by unrealistic wishes for cure that originate from the distress precipitated by a troubled or troubling teenager on these less controlled environments. That is, family members and school personnel see themselves as more limited in their ability to control a substance-abusing teenager. In their helplessness and relative lack of social leverage compared with the courts, they think that a program should "do something quick," "stop him (or her)," "let us get back to teaching," "let us have no more trouble," or "turn my kid back the way he (or she) used to be!"

5. Community mental health practitioners and consultants should understand the philosophy and jargon of a chemical dependence program; for example, they should be able to translate and integrate AA steps with diagnoses and treatment plans, with the phases of psychotherapy, with recovery, and with determining the appropriate level of care. Familiarity with Gorski and Miller's (1982) developmental model of recovery is essential. Some adaptation of motivation techniques of therapy applied to the treatment of adolescent substance abusers is needed, because group dynamics among disruptive adolescents may reinforce disruptive behavior rather than sobriety.

6. When presented with a difficult case, the community mental health practitioner and consultant should consider taking the opposite tack from the presenter to be seen as helpful, provocative, eclectic, and comprehensive. For example, if the counselor believes the patient has major depressive disorder and needs medication, the consultant might pay more attention to variables of developmental, chemical dependence, recovery, family dynamics, and milieu issues that could contribute to depression. This strategy can encourage a more comprehensive and effective treatment plan.

7. The community mental health practitioner and consultant must not get caught in the cross fire between proponents of the medical model and proponents of the chemical dependence/AA model of treatment. Both viewpoints have utility and are needed. Determine what can be used from each model to help resolve the patient's current crisis.

8. Chemical dependence and COD programs tend to operate frequently in a crisis mode precipitated by repeated, primitive, or chaotic behavior demonstrated by patients and family members. However, well-designed

programs have clearly outlined rules of conduct for patients and their families. Successful programs are usually considered to be governed by rules rather than by individuals. Generally, rules and consequences that affect the whole program tend to make teenagers with conduct disorders and chemical dependence protest that their individuality is being suppressed. Addicted teenagers tend to confuse the use of substances and the breaking of rules with the developmental task of forming an identity. Rule clarification and limit setting provide a predictable, coherent milieu and allow the teenagers to modify their view and feel safer from violence and exploitation.

9. An effective adolescent chemical dependence or COD program requires a critical mass of teenage patients who accept the merits of treatment and can maintain a positive therapeutic community. A commonly held belief in programs is that teenagers turn each other on to alcohol and other drugs and are therefore more effective in turning each other away from them. Those on the treatment-program staff, however, tend to take too much responsibility for the safety and effectiveness of the therapeutic milieu, for two reasons: 1) rapid patient turnover, which lowers the ratio of compliant to noncompliant patients; and 2) the natural law of teenagers and authority, which states that battles are inevitable.

The community mental health practitioner and consultant can take several measures to promote an effective milieu:

a. Expand the scope of a treatment program to include a continuum of services and allow transitioning teenagers in a less intensive treatment component to remain involved in the maintenance of the more intensive milieu, where trouble is more likely to brew.

b. Allow recovering teenagers in the treatment program to participate in the diagnostic evaluation sessions. In a structured group of an inpatient COD program for the initial evaluation, all peers can systematically ask very specific and pointed questions about the newcomer's problems. Peers are then given the opportunity to present their opinions about the new patient's level of substance use, psychosocial health, and need for help. For example, a female patient over time became adept at asking for valuable clinical information about substance use and the mental status of a new patient. This approach benefits all participants in the evaluation triad: the community mental health practitioner and consultant gather data faster and more accurately than from a resistant, angry, substance-abusing patient, because teenagers object less to inquiries from acceptable peers. New patients put their problems and recovery in perspective and pass through a significant institutionalized ritual of questioning to obtain a higher level in the therapeutic community. Finally, this process reinforces a key recovery principle that is especially supported in AA and NA: you help yourself by helping others.

c. Create patient government or committees to cooperate with the staff in overseeing the state of the program. Rules, rituals, consequences, and rewards have more meaning for recovery if everyone buys into them.

d. Involve more treatment-compliant but respected patients to keep order when a patient begins to "lose it" when limit setting and seclusion become options. Teenagers can be more effective than adults in calming and talking down their out-of-control peers. As an example, after his parents did not appear at a family therapy group, Billy refused to come out of his room, barricaded the door, threatened to trash his room and hit anyone who came near, and screamed, "I'd rather use drugs than deal with this crap." Conventionally, the staff would try to defuse the situation; set up consequences; or try to subdue, isolate, or seclude the patient. The psychiatrist would then be called to order seclusion and a psychotropic medication to calm the patient. Alternatively, the staff can find a peer or peers—who seem to have the most influence with the agitated teenager and the most to gain in keeping order in the program—to intervene. After hearing a few choice empathic words from a peer, Billy engaged in problem solving and found a way to save face. He agreed to a timeout and more support from his peers. A peer had de-escalated a situation that the staff might have overmanaged.

e. Do not become overly concerned with privacy as long as these peer counselors are still patients and have explicitly agreed to the program's rule on confidentiality.

10. An effective program needs to define how parents or guardians become involved in treatment. In too many programs, staff members back down from mandatory parental involvement and then are puzzled when the patients rebel against the staff. In this case, the staff has replaced the parents as the primary authority because the parents are not required to participate, examine themselves, and reassert their authority. Without mandatory parental involvement, the opportunity to intervene with parents who are impaired by substance abuse and other mental disorders is significantly reduced.

11. Ebbing and flowing levels of anxiety, depression, and impulsiveness from the staff reflect the current mental status of the treatment milieu or therapeutic community. Primitive defense mechanisms and behaviors of patients, dysfunctional behavior of families, and the pressures of managed care accountability are frequent elicitors of helplessness and hopelessness, turbulent emotions, erratic behavior, and illogical thought in the best of clinicians. When the staff are argumentative, uncooperative, blaming, or overly punitive or rejecting of patients and each other, look for the phenomenon of staff splitting. To be viewed as a leader, the community mental health practitioner and consultant must be more calm, empathic, rational, and adept at problem solving than the staff in the face of the clinical storms inherent in chemical dependence and COD programs.

12. Be wary of charismatic programs and leaders. The community mental health practitioner and consultant may discover considerable character flaws, including tunnel vision; an overbearing sense of self-righteousness (e.g., every client can be saved); possible unethical behavior; or an inability to differentiate between addiction, abuse, occasional self-destructive use, or infrequent use by a teenager going through a developmental phase or reacting to a family problem. These programs can dissolve if the leader leaves or acts too erratically. A practitioner might also be requested by an administrator to refrain from prescribing all psychotropics (sometimes called "mind-altering chemicals") for a youth who perhaps could benefit from an antidepressant.

13. The community mental health practitioner and consultant should expect to be an active and appropriately responsible participant in the admissions and discharge processes, whether he or she is the medical director, a consultant, or a practitioner. It is also important to create a reevaluation program or group for patients who are not responding to treatment. The practitioner can help the program define its vision, goals, and limitations and can help construct a policy and procedure manual aimed at maintaining a healthy culture for promoting healing regardless of who administers and leads the program.

14. Community mental health practitioners and consultants should expect their judgment and expertise to be challenged early on. Mental health practitioners will be envied, stereotyped, ignored, abhorred, and even admired. Some staff members of chemical dependence programs are recovering from addiction and have had unfortunate treatment experiences with mental health professionals. Some have little or inadequate mental health training. They may have extensive chemical dependence

training and a wealth of treatment experience. Some are quick and ea-
ger learners early in their careers or are "born therapists." The mental
health practitioner should maintain a stance of "Who knows what helps
a teenager recover?" Given the dearth of research, it is important to foster an active but respectful competition of ideas and interventions. To
enhance collegiality, chemical dependence counselors, psychiatric technicians, nurses, and others should be included in group or individual
sessions led or co-led by the psychiatrist. This inclusion provides for
staff education and interchange of ideas because it promotes integration
of the chemical dependence and mental health staff. Several of these
"raw recruits" may eventually move on to become trained as community mental health practitioners and consultants.

15. Community mental health practitioners and consultants should answer
these questions to orient themselves and to put any request by a staff
member in its proper context:

    a. How coherent is the program's mission and vision for encourag-
ing recovery from chemical dependence? How does it view continuity of services, CODs, mental health issues, medication issues,
and the like? Which patients can it evaluate and treat well?

    b. How organized are the clinical efforts regarding treatment plan-
ning and program construction? (A disorganized clinic cannot
heal a disorganized family or patient.)

    c. How well balanced and integrated are the traditional competing in-
terests of the chemical dependence staff and the mental health staff?

    d. Are psychiatrists viewed as team members or consultants?

Step 4: Study the Administrative Structure

Community mental health practitioners and consultants should make themselves aware of the health of any organization by asking the right questions:

• How well does the administration balance the provision of clinical services for
patients with the limitation of services to stay alive financially? Nonprofit, for-
profit, and public programs are all constrained by dollars. If a needed service
(e.g., aftercare or more-intensive outpatient services) does not exist, how can
a program really help its patients? To have a vibrant program, the directors
should be asking, "How do we find or create a service given our limits" rather
than saying, "We can't do it, because we can't afford it."

• How often does the administration include the viewpoint of psychiatrists
and other community mental health practitioners in making clinical deci-

sions with financial implications? (Traditional chemical dependence programs often err by not including psychiatrists who can comment on medical necessity and quality assurance issues.)

- Can this group survive the financial pressures of managed care, medical necessity criteria, and accountability?

- How well do the chief executive officer or administrative directors provide inspiration and leadership? How do they regard the need for psychiatric input, treatment, or consultation?

Step 5: Know Your Community

The youngsters eventually return to their schools and communities, where a certain level of substance abuse problems are either being addressed or ignored. The hard work done in treatment can be negated when a recovering teenager is tempted in the real world. It is important to ensure that supports in the community and school are part of the discharge treatment plan.

Step 6: Understand Your Role

Mental health professionals can assume the role of director, consultant, or practitioner. It may be helpful to keep in the mind the following points:

- Due to financial constraints and the time pressures of chemical dependence and COD programs, you may wear several hats in the same organization. Always clarify your roles when creating a contract, determine the intent of the staff and administration, and let them know that your function is changing. (Although hired as the medical director for a county governmental organization, this clinician had to shift roles constantly. As the medical director, I co-led the effort to create a system of care for substance-abusing adolescents. As a psychiatrist, I evaluated teenagers in the clinic and participated in treatment team meetings. As a consultant, I met with the directors of an intensive outpatient day school program to advise them on the improvement of the substance abuse component and consulted on the cases of several students in the program.) For legal and liability purposes, describe in writing your role and function.

- If you are an educator and trainer, expect requests to donate time setting up seminars or teaching about a psychiatric topic. A community mental health practitioner and consultant can help bring resources to a program. For example, pharmaceutical companies can provide funds for continuing education programs about CODs and can improve management by psychiatrists and the clinical staff of complex COD and other treatment-resistant cases; clinical staff members can feel more confident about their role and the psychiatrist's knowledge base in treating their clients.

Step 7: Understand How to Enter the System

The rules for entering a system differ little from general consultation, direct service, or medical/clinical directorship: the staff of most chemical dependence and COD programs respect community mental health practitioners and consultants who respect them and implicitly empathize with their distrust. The staff resent imperious or passive clinicians and respect those who can become "part of the gang." Mental health practitioners should make a point of attending continuing education programs on site or off site where the staff will appear. They should be involved in the admission and discharge processes to prevent inappropriate referrals and dismissals, as well as to preserve the effectiveness and integrity of the program.

Step 8: Become the Managed Care Expert

Community mental health practitioners and consultants should know the criteria for treatment at the different levels of a continuum of care (i.e., psychiatrists are most adept at synthesizing data, creating treatment plans, and justifying medical necessity). The practitioner should become the lead problem solver in determining the need for continuing care. This role will help the program determine its vision, which patients it has a chance of helping, and which should be referred.

Two tools are instrumental for advocating the best care for patients. The 2001 *ASAM (American Society of Addiction Medicine) Patient Placement Criteria for the Treatment of Substance-Related Disorders* offers detailed criteria about admission, continued stay, and discharge for adolescents. The American Association of Community Psychiatrists (1998) developed the Child and Adolescent Level of Care Utilization System (CALOCUS) for Psychiatric and Addiction Services. This system allows a treatment team to specify and quantify its decisions about placing a child or teenager at a specific level of care by incorporating criteria for levels of care with systems-of-care principles.

Step 9: Learn the Words and Take a Vacation "Somewhere"

See a production of *West Side Story* and listen to the words of the tune "Somewhere" that the lovers Tony and Maria sing. Community mental health practitioners and consultants need to keep their hope alive and make sure they take refreshing vacations to that essential "somewhere" so that they can return to the program renewed and ready for action. Chemical dependence and COD treatment are very stressful by nature and can lead to significant burnout. Take vacations to maintain hope and to creatively continue patients' effective treatment.

▌ CONCLUSIONS

Working in or consulting to an adolescent chemical dependence program can be both highly rewarding and extremely stressful. Implementing a series of steps as you enter this exciting and challenging area can help you acquire the insight, tools, and experience necessary to provide optimal, evidence-based care and to develop job satisfaction. Enjoying your work allows you to deliver the highest-quality care and to better assure yourself and the agency of your ability to continue such work for an extended period of productive time.

▌ REFERENCES

American Association of Community Psychiatrists: Child and Adolescent Level of Care Utilization System (CALOCUS) for Psychiatric and Addiction Services. Dallas, TX, American Association of Community Psychiatrists, 1998

American Society of Addiction Medicine: ASAM (American Society of Addiction Medicine) Patient Placement Criteria for the Treatment of Substance-Related Disorders, 2nd Edition, Revised. Chevy Chase, MD, American Society of Addiction Medicine, 2001

Gorski T, Miller M: Counseling for Relapse Prevention. Independence, MO, Independence Press, 1982

Winters KC (ed): Screening and Assessing Adolescents for Substance Use Disorders (Treatment Improvement Protocol [TIP] Series, 31; Publ No [SMA] 99-3282). Rockville, MD, Center for Substance Abuse Treatment, U.S. Department of Health and Human Services, 1999a

Winters KC (ed): Treatment of Adolescents With Substance Use Disorders (Treatment Improvement Protocol [TIP] Series, 32; Publ No [SMA] 99-3283). Rockville, MD, Center for Substance Abuse Treatment, U.S. Department of Health and Human Services, 1999b

▌ SUGGESTED READINGS

Bailey GW: Current perspectives on substance abuse in youth. J Am Acad Child Adolesc Psychiatry 28:151–162, 1989

Brook JS, Cohen P, Brook DW: Longitudinal study of co-occurring psychiatric disorders and substance use. J Am Acad Child Adolesc Psychiatry 37:322–330, 1998

Bukstein OG: Comorbidity and adolescent substance abuse, in Manual of Adolescent Substance Abuse Treatment. Edited by Estroff TW. Washington, DC, American Psychiatric Publishing, 2001, pp 69–89

Cohen PR: Treatment strategies with substance abusing adolescents, in Adolescent Substance Abuse and Dual Disorders. Edited by Jaffe SL. Child Adolesc Psychiatr Clin N Am 5:177-199, 1996

Jaffe SL, Simkin DR: Alcohol and drug abuse, in Child and Adolescent Psychiatry: A Comprehensive Textbook, 3rd Edition. Edited by Lewis M. Philadelphia, PA, Lippincott Williams & Wilkins, 2002, pp 895–911

Kastan J: Program development: organizing clinical innovations, in Dual Diagnosis: Evaluation, Treatment, Training, and Program Development. Edited by Solomon J, Zimberg S, Shollar E. New York, Plenum, 1993, pp 239–251

McLellan AT, Meyers K: Contemporary addiction treatment: a review of systems problems for adults and adolescents. Biol Psychiatry 56:764–770, 2004

Morral AR, McCaffrey DF, Ridgeway G: Effectiveness of community-based treatment for substance-abusing adolescents: 12-month outcomes of youths entering Phoenix Academy or alternative probation dispositions. Psychol Addict Behav 18:257–268, 2004

Newman L, Henry PB, DeRenzo P, et al: Intervention and student assistance: the Pennsylvania model. Journal of Chemical Dependency Treatment 2:145–162, 1989

O'Connell DF: Treating the high risk adolescent: a survey of effective programs and interventions. Journal of Chemical Dependency Treatment 2:39–70, 1989

Riggs P: Clinical approach to treatment of ADHD in adolescents with substance use disorders and conduct disorder. J Am Acad Child Adolesc Psychiatry 37:331–332, 1998

Riggs PD: Treating adolescents for substance abuse and comorbid psychiatric disorders. NIDA Science and Practice Perspectives 2(1):18–29, August 2003. Available at: http://www.drugabuse.gov/PDF/Perspectives/vol2no1/03Perspectives-Treating.pdf. Accessed May 19, 2005.

Schiff MM, Cavaiola AA: Adolescents at risk for chemical dependency: identification and prevention issues. Journal of Chemical Dependency Treatment 2:25–48, 1989

Silverman WH: Intervention strategies for the prevention of adolescent substance abuse. Journal of Adolescent Chemical Dependency 1:25–34, 1990

Wight JC: Family systems theory and adolescent substance abuse: a proposal for expanding the role of the school. Journal of Adolescent Chemical Dependency 1:57–76, 1990

Williams RJ, Chang SY: A comprehensive and comparative review of adolescent substance abuse treatment outcome. Clin Psychol 7:138–166, 2000

16 COMMUNITY RESIDENTIAL CARE PROGRAMS

Milton T. Fujita, M.D., M.H.A.

Valerie Arnold, M.D.

Residential treatment programs have developed within the continuum of community services for children and adolescents to meet the needs of those who have undergone multiple failed therapeutic interventions or for those who need a transition from a more restrictive to a less restrictive treatment setting as their treatment progresses. The Joint Commission on Accreditation of Healthcare Organizations (JCAHO) defines a residential program as a program that provides services to individuals who need a less structured environment than that of an inpatient program. Residential treatment programs have tremendous heterogeneity. Some serve specialized populations such as individuals with substance abuse, eating disorders, sexually inappropriate behaviors, or developmental disabilities. These programs vary in their degree of restrictiveness, ranging from supported living and small group homes with resident house parents to comprehensive residential treatment centers (RTCs) with a full range of professional services, including schools, secure units, and vocational training programs. The same principles may also apply to juvenile detention centers or boys' schools. The reader may wish to review work that provides a general overview of the history and a more detailed description of the functioning of such programs (Grigsby 2002; Lewis et al. 2002; Petti 2004). This chapter is directed to mental health professionals who are interested in working in or consulting to an agency that provides residential care and services.

Most residential programs have developed with the evolution of child welfare to meet the increasingly complex needs of children. Often staffed by individuals with varied experience in the mental health field, typical programs recruit mental health professionals as consultants or agency staff. Consultants might be asked to provide specialized input on a specific case or area of concern. For example, the administration or staff might seek help for a case in which making treatment decisions has created a rift between the staff and certain senior supervisors. The staff may be seeking additional professional input in the guise of training and supervision, whereas the administration may be seeking alternatives to its dilemma of maintaining staff cohesion. In this case, expert knowledge in the fields of child and adolescent psychiatry or related professions is what the clinical consultant is able to share (as opposed to being considered a consultant to the administration about human resource issues).

Several issues should be considered when deciding about working in a residential treatment program. The mental health consultant or employee will be expected to provide both information and direction in the treatment of the patients/residents, most of whom have complex histories and multiple treatment experiences. When considering joining an RTC or remaining involved with such a program, it is important to investigate the following critical areas:

• History of the agency and its planning process; the standing and structure of the agency
• Treatment philosophy of the agency
• Personnel issues
• Credentialing and related processes
• Personal growth and remuneration issues

These areas are applicable in relation to any public or private community agency. Before making a commitment of time and energy and accepting responsibilities and a position of authority, clarify each of these facets as they apply to yourself and the agency.

▮ THE COMMUNITY RESIDENTIAL CENTER OR GROUP HOME

History and Planning

Every agency has a history. Just as in a psychiatric evaluation of a new patient, you must gather relevant information about the development of the agency and its programs. The stature, structure, and evolution of the agency might be areas of particular interest. Financial instability, frequent change in leadership, or lack of change in leadership should lead you to take a cautious approach. Review of the long-range strategic plan and mission statement can give an idea about the future direction of the agency. Absence of a long-range strategic plan indicates the quality of leadership and may constitute a reason to reconsider pursuing the affiliation.

Organizational Credentials and Structure

Agency efforts in the painstaking exercise of developing a workable strategic plan with reasonable goals are usually seen as a plus—but are the goals and direction chosen compatible with your own ideas of treatment? Does the mission statement reflect acceptable parameters within which you will be able to provide services (e.g., whether the agency is affiliated with a church organization, whether the mission statement and strategic plan are acceptable guides for you)?

The agency's overall treatment philosophy becomes an important guide to how far you are willing to nurture the relationship. Your ability to combine the agency's treatment philosophy and your own will be crucial in determining your role in the care of the children. The agency's standing in the professional community should provide a sense of its ability to collaborate with other local and statewide services. For example, the types of children who are referred for residential and group home programs require availability of multiple resources. Access to, coordination of, and integration of such resources often require cooperation and collaboration between several entities, either local or statewide.

Organizational competence and integration are also reflected in the types of accreditation attained by the agency. An agency that seeks and maintains accreditation from JCAHO or the Council on Accreditation should be taken seriously. It has invested significant amounts of staff time and agency funds into upgrading the program to meet national quality standards. Maintaining accreditation requires the agency to monitor multiple aspects of the treatment process. In the era of the managed-care mentality, these accrediting guidelines are often the basis for financial reimbursement through state and private payer agency contracts. Likewise, affiliation with the local United Way indicates significant attention to accountability and the possible commitment of additional resources. United Way funding can be significant to many smaller agencies in which financial stability is shaky. Moreover, the additional networking with other community programs broadens the scope of available resources for children served by the agency.

For agencies that rely heavily on donations, the structure of the board of directors is especially critical. A prospective employee or consultant should ask for a list (often found on the agency letterhead) of board members and if possible some information about their roles in the community. Leadership provided by an active, informed board of respected community leaders enhances the agency's stature and financial backing for developing and maintaining good treatment programs. If many of the names are not familiar, seek more information from outside the agency. A board is effective only to the degree of its oversight. Questions about the frequency of meetings may be helpful in determining its investment.

Communication between the board and the administration is crucial for an agency's success. Depending on your potential role or position in the agency, meeting with the board chairman or a member of the board may be a useful way of learning the board's point of view, the members' commitment to the agency, and their degree of involvement in the agency's operation. Potential employees or consultants may wish to assimilate this information with that gained from meeting with administrative staff. A committed board is an outstanding asset, but a board engaged in day-to-day operations suggests basic problems in the agency's functioning and stability.

The final and most important aspect of the agency's structure is its organization chart. The chain of command is crucial to how major decisions are made and implemented. These decisions eventually affect the treatment process. Employees or consultants will want to have some sense of the manner in which their recommendations will be conveyed to and accepted by those in charge. This structure and process may determine how and when you would share information and recommendations to improve organizational performance. The organization chart can provide information to guide monitoring of the organization's functioning.

How major communications are shared within an organization and among the personnel is especially important in residential programs. In meeting and discussing various issues with management and staff, patterns of internal communication should emerge. Quality of care, morale, and overall agency functioning are dependent on the extent and effectiveness of communication with the staff by management and the perception by staff members that they are heard by management. If the staff perceives that they are not being heard by management, you may be faced with several dilemmas. For example, as a member of the mental health professional staff, you may be unofficially designated to champion their cause for recognition. Your stature as a physician, psychiatrist, clinical psychologist, social worker, or nurse may be seen by certain members of the staff as a reason to designate or identify you as the spokesperson to carry their concerns to management. The staff may overestimate your influence because they believe that you understand their role "in the trenches" and that you are respected by management. You will need to determine whether you feel comfortable accepting such a role and managing situations when significant dissonance exists over particular issues in light of the agency's culture and structure. Most agencies have members with a vested interest in maintaining the status quo who will present issues that serve as temporary barriers to anyone with new ideas. How you handle such issues may determine your effectiveness in working within or consulting to the agency or in directing treatment teams or agency components at higher administrative levels. As a consultant, you will be given as much information as the staff may feel is safe until they can determine how much trust their leaders place in your views and recommendations. The more highly influential you are perceived to be, the more likely it is that you may become designated to carry the cause to the administration. As a consultant, you are an advocate for improving services and access to those in need. Distinguishing between the role of champion for those with whom you consult and such an advocacy role for the residents and their families can be a challenge.

You should contact the state trade organization of residential care providers to learn if the residential program is a member, its degree of involvement, and how it compares to similar state programs. These organizations provide critical lobbying efforts, education, coordination, and collaboration in providing quality care.

Treatment Philosophy

Agencies dealing with residential care of emotionally disturbed children and adolescents have altered their mode of treatment over the years. As the filtering process identifies the more severely affected children as being in more acute need and more money is relegated to their care, established programs have had to adjust and readjust treatment strategies to meet those needs within limitations necessary to maintain financial viability. Meetings with the agency directors can help determine the basic treatment philosophy and how it meets all or part of the children's needs. Is there evidence that most patients move to a less restrictive treatment program or even back to their families? Or do more residents have longer stays than are expected or accepted by community standards?

Certain guideposts can help you judge an agency's overall effectiveness and ability to carry out its mission. The agency's policies, procedures, and functioning in the following areas are critical to care and are good indicators of its quality:

- Group homes require fewer staff members and available services on site.
- Agencies designated as an RTC or a comprehensive RTC must be able to provide a full range of services on campus and require a well-coordinated

system with cooperation from top to bottom with a significant number of professional staff members.

- The span of cooperation is more diffuse when an agency uses off-campus services (e.g., educational services), assumes the role of parent, and must represent the children's interests in their participation in regular school activities and extracurricular programs.
- Cooperation and coordination are even more essential in treating students who require special education services.
- The concept of providing a continuum of care should exist to a certain extent beyond the educational program.
- The treatment process should emphasize goals to assist residents in continuing their emotional and educational growth outside the agency's scope.
- A quality assurance program should be in place.

Participation in treatment team meetings is the quickest and best way to gain a sense of the agency's overall philosophy. How the meeting is conducted and how staff members participate can be telling details. The degree of representation from all the disciplines that have contact with the child provides a sense of the depth of treatment. An understanding of how treatment decisions are made can provide perspective into how you may fit into the system. The level of expertise of the staff reflects the degree to which the administration is committed to good treatment. You may wish to use your experience gained during or after training of well-run teams or agencies to compare and contrast the quality of team functioning. Monitoring various campus activities is essential for guiding the staff in providing service.

Variance in quality assurance sophistication among agencies is usually dependent on the level of service and the agency administration's commitment to self-monitoring and maintaining accreditation. In briefly reviewing the quality assurance plan, check the areas being monitored, the type of information being gathered, and how the information is collected. Although the data may be collected and collated electronically, the staff must provide the information by entering it into computers or completing forms. An indicator of ineffective communication may be shown in staff discontent arising from time-consuming data collection tasks when there is heavy demand for them to provide direct services and fulfill other duties.

Your Role

There are multiple roles within group home or RTC settings that a psychiatrist or other mental health professional can assume. Each role has a different level of responsibility and liability, as described in Chapter 1, "Working

Within Communities." A *consultant* typically makes recommendations but is not responsible for the direct implementation of the treatment. In contrast, being in a *supervisory* role carries the responsibility not only for making suggestions regarding care but also for seeing that the treatment is initiated. In such a role, you assume responsibility and liability for the decisions made by those whom you supervise. You may contract to provide *direct services* to agencies either on-site or off-site and on an on-call, scheduled, or emergency basis. Your responsibility for direct services such as evaluations, psychotherapy, or medication management to individual patients is no less than if you were in private practice. Lastly, an *administrative role* requires that you participate in making major decisions within the agency and may expose you to additional areas of liability.

These roles affect agencies—which may or may not have previously had the benefit of receiving input from psychiatric or other mental health professionals in making decisions—and are associated with major pitfalls you may encounter such as admission and discharge policies. Decisions already made by the chief executive officer, program director, or someone influenced by a board member may be presented to you as an "option for your consideration" to gain your approval. The intent may only be to add expert weight to a policy or procedure, but it is critical to have open dialogue around such issues to avoid misunderstandings that place you in a no-win situation. Other potential pitfalls are taking on the supervisor role when your contract is for consultation or without the assigned authority to ensure that your recommendations are implemented. As noted above under "Organizational Credentials and Structure," knowledge of the agency's organization chart is imperative if you are to function effectively. For example, many residents in RTCs or group homes do not have a psychiatrist or other physician assigned to them.

Admission and discharge decisions made without input from a physician (or, when applicable, a psychologist or psychiatrist) raise concerns about malpractice liability and responsibility to third-party payers (e.g., Medicaid). Delineation of roles and responsibilities ensures that everyone is better able to understand and meet his or her responsibilities:

> On her weekly consultation visit to an RTC, a child psychiatrist saw a few patients and provided pharmacotherapy. She learned that a resident had been decertified when a nonclinician told the primary therapist to discharge the patient over the weekend. The resident was taking no medications, and the records indicated that the order to discharge was verbal.

This case raises some important considerations:

- How patient discharge decisions are made and who has the authority to make those decisions should be clearly communicated to all staff members. In this case, was a nonclinical person authorized to make that decision, or was it intended as a suggestion?

- Treatment plans should specify the discharge date that was formally discussed by the treatment team.

- In many settings, seemingly unimportant orders (e.g., diets, issuance of passes to patients, continuation of medication) are indicated as verbal orders without a physician being called. Physicians should determine when and if this is happening at their institutions.

Personnel Issues

Accredited agencies have readily available job descriptions for their employees that clearly identify required qualifications and responsibilities of the individual versus responsibilities of the agency. Job descriptions for mental health professionals are often generic. (Please see the chapters in Part 2, "The Core Mental Health Professionals," for details that can be included in the description.) Roles and responsibilities should be clarified in interviews with agency personnel. Retain notes of your meetings with agency members to compare opportunities and as a guide in reviewing your contract. It would be prudent to have an attorney review the final contract before you sign it.

Contracts range from generic to highly specific. All contracts should include details such as starting date, duration of contract, scope of service (which may or may not include being on call), specifics of compensation, required malpractice and liability coverage, and conditions that outline cancellation of the contract. The noncompete clause is particularly controversial, because it can limit your ability to practice in the community if you leave the agency under certain conditions. Decide whether such a clause with mutually acceptable parameters should be included.

Specific issues surrounding compensation should be clearly stated. Are you salaried or paid on an hourly basis? If paid hourly, are you paid to attend to administrative issues or attend meetings other than those directly related to patient care? Are you expected to be on call? If so, is it by telephone or in person? How is your time to be monitored if your involvement is not the same each time? Agencies often contract for a specific number of hours per week or per month. However, occasions may arise when you may be required to provide extra hours. How will the extra time of work be resolved? Likewise, are you expected to bill the agency for your services with details of dates and time worked?

In today's managed care environment, the billing process is a critical consideration that consumes considerable resources. The following questions are highly germane to whether the agency can continue to fund your position:

- Are the services you provide part of an all-inclusive rate covered under a Medicaid Rehabilitation Option, or do they fall under another category?
- If you are to charge fees, will the agency bill third-party payers for the services you provide, or are you expected to carry out this task?
- If you are salaried, will your time be distributed equitably to meet both administrative and clinical demands?
- Are you expected to generate a percentage of your salary, or is your salary based on a percentage of what you generate through clinical work?
- Are there financial consequences for failing to meet a certain income, productivity quota, or quality monitor? If so, are the consequences of the resultant rewards or penalties specified?

The agency person who monitors or evaluates your performance and to whom you report should be identified. It is prudent to meet with this person to assess your ability to work together. Also of concern are any ancillary issues discussed during negotiations that fail to materialize (e.g., secretarial support was promised but was not included in the written contract):

> A psychiatrist was hired to consult on a half-time basis to an RTC. Several months after he began his consultation, the secretary who had been assigned to transcribe his notes was promoted, and there was no attempt to fill the vacancy.

Such a situation, rife for ongoing conflict and hostility, can be easily avoided by anticipating such occurrences through your earlier efforts to understand the agency's mode of functioning and, if necessary, making written provisions.

This example highlights a difference in technology utilization between some public and private community agencies that provide mental health treatment. Some agencies expect notes to be dictated or typed to meet the requirements of regulatory and accrediting bodies. Others accept handwritten notes as long as they include the date and time written. Clarifying the agency's expectations and degree of support for the more technologically advanced options should be a major focus of negotiations, particularly for the busy clinician with poor handwriting skills.

Continuing education is crucial for quality of care and to maintain the morale of mental health professionals. Expectations of both the professional and the agency, including time off and compensation for continuing education, should be articulated early on. Psychiatrists and other mental health professionals too often depend on the magical thinking that if they work hard and provide quality service, they will be rewarded and reimbursed properly.

Working in the public sector, particularly with community RTCs, can provide a high degree of job satisfaction. But just as you set financial expectations with your patients, you should do the same with your employer. The caveat is to be certain that issues of importance to your functioning, remuneration, responsibility, and authority are clearly defined and included as appropriate in written contracts. The time spent in learning about the agency should direct your attention to the critical issues that can influence the degree of success and satisfaction you achieve from working in or consulting to the agency.

Credentialing Process

The number of credentials you will be asked to provide an employer (and often to any managed care entity for whom the agency provides service) is amazing. There is the standard request for copies of your state license and board certificate (and for child and adolescent psychiatrists, U.S. Drug Enforcement Administration and both state and federal controlled substance registration certificates); evidence of malpractice insurance coverage; and Medicare and Medicaid provider numbers. There may be additional requirements for proof of membership in health maintenance organizations' preferred provider networks, managed care organizations, and hospital staffs, depending on the level and sophistication of the agency's funding stream. As quality management becomes integrated into the process of medicine and human services, psychiatrists and other mental health professionals will be expected to be on board. Become familiar with the process and terminology of managed care programs as soon as possible. Understanding the concept and terminology will help you assess whether the performance objectives established by your agency are reasonable and attainable with the available resources. The clearer these issues are to you, the more job satisfaction you should experience and the less conflict you should have with your agency as well as with the children and families you serve. This understanding should clarify any performance measures that may be in place that could affect your functioning and the agency's ability to obtain compensation for your work and that of staff members whom you supervise.

Considering related issues may also be worthwhile. For example, psychiatrists might consider that payers are cautious about including an RTC as a network provider because of the possibility of opening a door for the customers they insure. Agencies may want to take advantage of the relative ease with which physicians can join a managed care panel and may be willing to process the voluminous paperwork required to join some networks. However, psychiatrists risk removal from these panels if the billing under the psychiatrist's name is perceived as being excessive. This consequence needs careful assessment for any professional that may be involved. Once removed from a panel, a physician generally has great difficulty getting reinstated.

Professional Growth Issues

During training, you were able to balance your reading and clinical learning experiences with service provided to your patients. You had supervisors whom you regularly met with. Such opportunities for growth are not as readily available when working in group homes or RTCs, especially those without university affiliations. The minimal degree of professional involvement impedes residential programs' ability to mutually interact with and enrich colleagues. You may want to consider the following items to enhance your professional growth:

- Determine how important continuing education is to you.
- Investigate the support and the type of in-service training and continuing education that other staff members receive for attending educational programs and for earning the continuing education credits required by some licensing and certifying boards.
- Find other opportunities for personal growth, including meeting with other professionals in the community to network about the residents and their needs, working with advocacy and self-help groups, interacting with professional organizations and policy makers, and consulting with senior clinicians from your discipline.
- Seek opportunities to collaborate with researchers, educators, and clinicians from universities regarding program evaluation or research.

Access by support staff to in-service training that you conduct or in which you participate may also be crucial to your job performance and satisfaction. Training the staff at an RTC or group home can be a challenging and rewarding task that can enhance your competence and job satisfaction.

▮ CONCLUSIONS

In deciding whether to join or continue to work in or with a group home or RTC, consider how successful you will be in the role. Take time to meet with administrative staff, treatment team staff, and, when appropriate, members of the board of directors before making the decision. Will it be possible for you to blend with the agency's culture, to be accepted by the other disciplines, and to share a common view of the residents' best interests? Psychiatrists and other mental health professionals are being asked with increasing frequency to provide better services with fewer resources for sicker individuals. This reality highlights the vital importance that your basic personal, fiscal, and professional needs be met and that both agency management and professional staff members have compatible views on availability, authority, responsibility, rewards, and goals.

The agency's involvement with managed care organizations is likely to accelerate over the next few years. Administrators of RTCs, group homes, and other organizations that are integrated within a continuum of care may become concerned about the intrusion of managed care into their system. Compelled to modify their behavior, RTCs that customarily employed extended lengths of stay are planning quicker transitions back into the community and are using less restrictive interventions. Clinicians are under considerable pressure to work fewer hours while managing severely disturbed youths during briefer stays in hospitals and residential centers. These seeming conflicts complete the picture of the system of residential care that seeks dedicated professionals who are quick thinkers with lots of energy and a capacity for active problem solving. These issues are germane to those considering employment within a residential setting and to those contemplating the advisability of remaining in a system in which they feel valued and productive.

The ongoing movement toward a continuum-of-care system will lead agencies to develop novel strategies to meet multiple needs. Many residential care agencies will join with public-sector managed care organizations to develop innovative approaches to assessment and treatment by employing a model of blended funding or decategorization of funds and less-restrictive resource sharing. The next several years should witness advances in partnerships that can barely be imagined at this time. You have an opportunity to join in this evolution of ideas and idealism as a staff member, supervisor, administrator, or consultant to a residential care program.

▍ REFERENCES

Grigsby RK: Consultation with foster care homes, group homes, youth shelters, domestic violence shelters, and Big Brothers and Big Sisters programs, in Child and Adolescent Psychiatry: A Comprehensive Textbook, 3rd Edition. Edited by Lewis M. Philadelphia, PA, Lippincott Williams & Wilkins, 2002, pp 1393–1398

Lewis M, Summerville JW, Graffagnino PN: Residential treatment, in Child and Adolescent Psychiatry: A Comprehensive Textbook, 3rd Edition. Edited by Lewis M. Philadelphia, PA, Lippincott Williams & Wilkins, 2002, pp 1095–1103

Petti TA: Milieu treatment: inpatient, partial, residential, in Textbook of Child and Adolescent Psychiatry, 3rd Edition. Edited by Wiener J, Dulcan M. Washington, DC, American Psychiatric Publishing, 2004, pp 1055–1074

17 WORKING WITH ADVOCACY GROUPS

Claire Griffin-Francell, C.N.S./P.M.H., M.S.N.

In recent years, families of children and adolescents with serious emotional disturbance (SED) have joined for support and advocacy to improve mental health services and end discrimination. Although slow at times, significant progress has brought professionals and advocates together to speak out for better services and supports. The purpose of this chapter is to help psychiatric professionals understand their role in working successfully with advocacy groups.

■ UNDERSTANDING THE TERRITORY

First, practitioners need persistence and patience to engage with advocacy groups and coalitions. The major challenges are to find a balance between the roles of provider and advocate and to acknowledge that each role has its own traditions, rules, and sanctions. Partnership implies equality, which historically is rarely found in these two groups. Few mental health professionals actually engage in pro bono service, which is a selfless commitment to advancing best practices in professional life; but when they do volunteer, they often find that the energy of advocates becomes contagious and can renew a career burdened by responsibility.

The author wishes to acknowledge the assistance of Edward G. Francell Jr., M.S.W., in the preparation of this chapter.

Psychiatric providers often need to prepare for a lengthy education in developing relationships with advocates and must discard outdated knowledge and beliefs. A provider must first understand the crucial relationship between public policy and political advocacy. A highly effective way to learn about this relationship is to experience a field placement that includes working with advocacy groups. Most practitioners begin advocacy relationships without this experience and thus may become discouraged in trying to develop satisfying and effective partnerships.

Before outlining the skills required to overcome this discouragement and work successfully with advocates, it is important to review the history of children's mental health advocacy, an effort similar to other societal movements such as those for civil rights, women's suffrage, and disability rights. A summary of some major milestones in children's mental health advocacy is presented in Table 17–1.

Past Advocates for Children

Concerned advocates helped to formulate a proclamation at the 1930 White House Conference on Child Health and Protection stating that emotionally disturbed children had the same right to develop normally as other children. In 1969, the congressionally created Joint Commission on the Mental Health of Children issued a report identifying significant problems facing American children and calling for development of a national child advocacy system. The response was mostly symbolic, and no significant change followed in the next decade.

In 1982, educational researcher Jane Knitzer published *Unclaimed Children: The Failure of Public Responsibility to Children and Adolescents in Need of Mental Health Services,* which systematically highlighted the profound failure of public systems to effectively treat children with severe psychiatric and behavioral disorders. The book brought together professionals and families along with community leaders to inform federal and state legislators about their responsibilities. Congress responded in 1984 by establishing the Child and Adolescent Service System Program (CASSP), which was designed to create organized systems of care for children with SED.

CASSP allocated funds to state mental health departments through the National Institute of Mental Health. However, inadequate appropriations permitted creation of few local systems. State governments were expected to enlarge and continue federal efforts without citizen support for additional funding. State and federal authorities became experts at a fiscal shell game, in which each side tried to shift the cost of treatment to the other side. Despite the problems of CASSP, it remained a significant start in establishing a basic framework for a rational child and adolescent mental health system.

TABLE 17–1. Major milestones in children's mental health advocacy

Year	Action
1930	White House Conference on Child Health and Protection
1969	Federal report *Crisis in Child Mental Health* released (Joint Commission on the Mental Health of Children 1969)
1982	*Unclaimed Children* published by Jane Knitzer (1982)
1984	Child and Adolescent Service System Program established
2003	Paul Wellstone Mental Health Equitable Treatment Act introduced in Congress

In 1997, Senators Pete Domenici (R–New Mexico) and Paul Wellstone (D–Minnesota) sponsored a budget reconciliation bill amendment giving children and adults with psychiatric disorders full parity in health insurance. Business and insurance groups fought the amendment, whereas family advocates aggressively supported it. A watered-down compromise did little to address inadequate mental health insurance and was mostly a symbolic victory. The fight moved to state legislatures, producing parity laws, many of which contained large loopholes that rendered them virtually useless. Family advocates garnered support in both the House and Senate in 2001 for a much more comprehensive parity bill, but it was defeated in a congressional conference committee. After the death of Senator Wellstone in 2002, the bill was reintroduced in Congress as the Paul Wellstone Mental Health Equitable Treatment Act (2003).

Major Areas Where Advocacy Is Needed

Historically, families of psychiatrically disabled children have interacted with two or more of four primary systems: the educational system, the mental health system, the juvenile justice system, and the welfare system. Each system overlaps the others, with many areas available for advocacy opportunity (Figure 17–1).

Each system presents challenges, but even the strongest of parents with disabled children can feel overwhelmed from the strains of dealing with the tests these systems convey. Before the emergence of the advocacy movement, parents' preferences regarding treatment or their limited financial resources were only rarely taken into account. Primarily due to inertia and stasis, change in social systems was often resisted and avoided. As advocates learned more about problems with these systems, they began reaching out to new allies.

Mental health

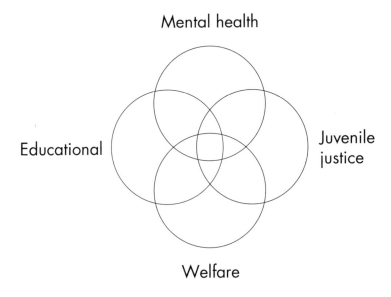

Educational

Juvenile justice

Welfare

FIGURE 17–1.   Interacting systems in children's mental health: areas for potential advocacy.

Professionals acknowledge that some peers still hold hostile and blameful attitudes toward families—but also recognize that some families have unreasonable expectations. Families vary enormously in their composition, culture, education, and financial resources. Noted psychiatrist and advocate E. Fuller Torrey said, "The only thing families may have in common is that you have an ill relative" (personal communication, 1997). This applies to advocacy groups as well. Professionals will move beyond avoiding problems or labeling advocates as antiprofessionals or troublemakers if they view parents' anger as a normal response to tragedy instead of a personal attack.

The Fragmentation of State Mental Health Care Delivery Systems

In the past, families often encountered underfunded, nonstandardized non-systems of care that appeared confusing, chaotic, and often exploitive. In the 1980s, many private, for-profit psychiatric hospitals were created to optimize revenues, with quality of care being relegated to a token consideration. Accountability in children's mental health through the adoption of meaningful and measurable outcomes was nonexistent. Although many clinicians focused on the immediate goals of diagnosis, stabilization, and change, administrators concerned themselves primarily with costs.

After exhausting private insurance, families were forced to turn to a fragmented, overworked, and understaffed public mental health system. Some common public mental health system realities included long hospital waiting lists and extraordinarily fragmented services. A particularly repugnant practice involved asking families to relinquish custody in order for a child to receive treatment, often producing extreme guilt and despair in parents. Change has been slow in these areas. One bright spot is that parental rights in treatment decisions have recently begun to be acknowledged and taken seriously in some areas.

The Failure of Past Preprofessional Educational Programs

When advocates started to look at mental health training programs in universities, they found many problems. Standard curricula included psychoanalytically oriented models that promoted distance from families. Emerging biological and genetic etiologies were absent or barely mentioned. The standard family therapy model covertly blamed families for damaging children and viewed families as toxic agents. Some families participated in "re-parenting" programs that charged insurance carriers high fees for their treatments, which sometimes utilized unorthodox and bizarre methods. Enormous amounts of time and money were spent trying to find and correct family flaws through psychodynamic therapies, usually with little or no success. Some observers concluded that much of what passed for treatment constituted no more than educated guesses, and often wrong guesses at that.

Knowledge Dissemination: The Advocates' Mission

In the late 1970s, brain imaging and radioactive scanning technologies began to uncover the physical basis of behavioral disorders. A paradigm shift in treatment models coincided with increasing knowledge of brain dysfunction and the hope that these new insights would aid the understanding and treatment of childhood psychiatric disorders.

Gradually, content about families and treatment changed to reflect this awareness. When autism research uncovered a biological basis for delay in brain development, compassion for families of autistic children started to replace blame. Outcomes of new psychiatric research helped balance treatment between biological and psychological interventions, and there was less reliance on talk therapy as a sole intervention. The use of medications to treat mental disorders had not fared well in the public eye, with many exaggerated and sometimes fabricated stories of methylphenidate (Ritalin) abuse being most prominent. A focus on outcomes led to the development of treatment guidelines for both biological and psychological therapies. The introduction of an evidence-based treatment philosophy strengthened the new partnership model of sharing responsibility and decision making between parent and provider and helped both parents and providers make decisions truly in the best interest of the child.

▌ ADVOCACY IN THE HUMAN SERVICES SYSTEM

Advocacy in the Educational Environment

For years, school systems exhausted the parents of disabled children, because no legal means existed to hold local school authorities responsible for educating this population—and the schools simply refused to serve these children. In 1975, Congress passed the Education for All Handicapped Children Act (EHA; P.L. 94-142), requiring every disabled child to receive an Individual Education Plan, a customized blueprint to secure a free and appropriate education in the least restrictive environment possible. Local school boards rethought their obligations to disabled children and their families, and coalitions of parents, legal advocates, and progressive educators worked hard to hold school systems accountable.

How to integrate children with physical disabilities was obvious, with school systems providing for mobility, medications, and other needs. Children with psychiatric and behavioral disorders, however, were a very different story. The 1997 congressional battle over amending the EHA—which was then renamed the Individuals With Disabilities Education Act (P.L. 105-17)—demonstrated how reluctant the public was to accept psychiatric impairments as true disabilities. The most troublesome issue for teachers surrounded safety: the presence of children susceptible to violently acting out challenged the concept of the classroom as the least restrictive environment. These problems demanded a creative response that was sensitive to everyone's rights, especially the right of children to receive effective psychiatric treatment. The outcome of containing violent behavior would allow students to learn and teachers to teach. Coalitions of teachers, parent advocates, and expert professionals began to work together to overcome this problem.

Nationally, coalitions of advocacy groups joined together to effect change. In the 1980s, the Association for Children With Learning Disabilities (ACLD) emerged as a voice for disabled children, initially monitoring implementation of laws regarding education of neurologically disabled children. With chapters in 50 states, the ACLD engaged in individual case and system advocacy. The ACLD—now known as the Learning Disabilities Association of America—worked to bring about change in university schools of education, which prepare special education teachers as well as regular classroom teachers.

The Juvenile Justice System: A Challenge for the Strong

Children with SED often experience legal trouble; however, juvenile justice systems mostly operate under a philosophy based on punishment and the protection of society. Out-of-control children who act out brain dysfunction through antisocial behavior often wind up in juvenile detention facilities, where treatment is scarce or nonexistent. The lack of mental health treatment resources is a continuing source of frustration to criminal justice personnel, families, and concerned citizens. As psychiatric hospitals have been downsized, the numbers of jail and prison inmates with psychiatric impairments have correspondingly increased. The actual prevalence of psychiatric disorders among incarcerated youths varies widely but is significant (Teplin et al. 2002). The statistics highlight the interrelations between mental disorders and children at risk for legal problems.

In the early 1990s, mental health, correctional, and law enforcement professionals joined family members and consumers for a conference on juvenile justice and children's mental health sponsored by the National Coalition for Mental and Substance Abuse Health Care in the Justice System, Community Action for the Mentally Ill Offender, and the National Institute of Corrections. The conference helped formulate amendments to the Juvenile Justice and Delinquency Prevention Act of 1974 (P.L. 93-415). The new law, Juvenile Justice and Delinquency Prevention Reauthorization Act (P.L. 102-506), was enacted in 1993. It provided federal assistance at the state, local and private levels. The National Coalition developed a state policy design to formulate solutions to the problems of juvenile justice and children's mental health. Across the country, the pace of change toward improving services in juvenile justice facilities currently is directly correlated with the strength of the local advocacy movement.

Helping Improve Services in Juvenile Justice

In every community, there are many ways for mental health professionals to assist child mental health advocates with juvenile justice issues. Advocates need help educating police officers (at police academies, for example) and sheriffs, as well as staffs at juvenile detention facilities. Judges and lawyers need information to understand which disorders constitute SED, their proper treatment, and which behaviors signal the need for treatment.

Every large city needs advocates to help organize and run a coalition for children with brain disorders in the criminal justice system. The presence of a psychiatric professional on the advocacy team can lend credibility to efforts and can open closed doors. For example, in Birmingham, Alabama, the local affiliate of the National Alliance for the Mentally Ill (NAMI) was instrumental in organizing a successful coalition of family members, judges, and criminal justice officers. It serves as a resource for other groups and shares information at minimal cost. Numerous opportunities exist for psychiatric professionals to organize or support coalitions by using their skills, knowledge, and influence to advocate for troubled children. The credibility of both academic and community-based professionals can add to the efforts of parent groups and can make a real difference in outcomes.

The Welfare System: A Work Needing Progress

The needs of a disabled child sometimes prevent a parent from working outside the home or severely limit his or her ability to provide the necessities of life to the family, often resulting in the need to seek public assistance. Many parents of children with SED perceive that overburdened state medical assistance and welfare programs are more sympathetic to children who are blind, retarded, deaf, or mobility impaired. Families that are struggling to survive often cannot respond to efforts of psychiatric practitioners if their immediate priorities are food, shelter, and clothing. (See Chapter 12, "Foster Care Programs," for a view from the foster family perspective.)

▌ GETTING STARTED IN ADVOCACY

There are many opportunities for professionals to make a difference through advocacy. It is important to start by researching advocacy groups you have admired or noticed in the past. Think about why a particular advocacy group caught your attention, considering such factors as its leadership, people's personalities, outcomes achieved, and strategies used. Once one or two interesting groups are identified, begin research on the organizations by browsing their Web sites, requesting their literature, or speaking with members. It is often helpful to conduct an environmental scan of the organization, asking key questions to establish compatibility and to gauge the group's effectiveness (Table 17–2).

TABLE 17–2. Environmental scan of advocacy organizations

Philosophy

Is the organization's mission and work compatible with your beliefs?

Can you compromise on any points you may disagree on?

What books does the group promote? Are the authors well known and respected in their field?

Peers

Have any of your colleagues heard about the organization?

Have they heard about the group's impression of providers? What do they think? What do you think?

What contact have they had with the group? What was their experience of this contact?

Time commitment

How much time do you want to contribute to the organization?

Are there opportunities outside your work hours to contribute?

Are you required to receive approval from your current employer to participate in the group?

Getting Involved With the Right Group

After examining possible groups, look at potential barriers to your involvement, then examine how to overcome them. Is the group's office nearby geographically? Are there a national office, a state office, and a local group? Is it possible to attend a local group meeting or travel to a national or state conference or to state capitals to lobby legislators? Is associate membership status available to professionals, or full membership with voting privileges?

Organizations often welcome a professional's help. Professionals can help with various committee efforts: fund-raising, public policy, education, government affairs, public relations, and so forth. Perhaps the advocacy group needs a liaison to the provider's professional association. After evaluating your personal values and professional goals, it is time to choose the best method of involvement.

Defining Your Role

A good way to begin contact is by arranging to meet the local or state president or board members. It is important to size up designated leaders so that you can determine possible roles in the organization (e.g., crisis resource, speaker, newsletter article writer, or legislative committee member) and define limits. You may have to emphasize a desired role. The group's executive director can help you define your limits to the group—often a challenging and delicate matter. Most advocacy groups, despite negative experiences, welcome involvement by professionals. They will usually accept the role the professional defines.

Making a Commitment

Attend a meeting of the board of directors to meet leaders and learn about advocacy issues. Disclosing that you are a consumer or that one of your relatives is a consumer will quickly establish your credibility. Pay your membership dues as soon as possible. Request copies of the organization's brochures, place them in your office, and give them to peers. Do not commit to what cannot be delivered, and do not backtrack on involvement unless there is a legitimate reason to do so. An honest commitment will result in acceptance. Try to overlook members' quirks, flaws, and lack of knowledge and focus instead on their energy and passion.

An overview of the steps for becoming involved with an advocacy group is presented in Figure 17–2.

Advocates' Expectations About Professionals' Involvement

During interviews with child advocate leaders, clear expectations have surfaced about what professionals can contribute. Referral of families to advocacy groups is a high priority. Family testimonies include statements such as "The group saved my life" and "I felt less like a failure." Advocates also appreciate assistance in fund-raising, a pressing need of many organizations. Professionals can also sponsor joint conferences on children's issues and can open their workplace facilities for conferences.

Joint appearances at public meetings and forums are other ways to help. Advocates may want professionals to appear jointly with them at parent-teacher association meetings to speak about children's needs, or they may want professionals to help them educate juvenile justice judges and lawyers about psychiatric disorders. Advocates who feel that professionals can help them develop relationships and prestige with community leaders often regard such professionals as door openers. Leading advocates may want professionals to ask their state and national professional organizations to develop position papers on certain issues (e.g., a need for children to have access to newer, more effective medications). Advocates often say that professional groups rarely stick their collective necks out by writing public position papers; such public positions are badly needed.

However, advocates also expect professionals to take direction from the advocacy group and to realize that families have credibility because of their experiences. They expect professionals to use nontechnical language so fam-

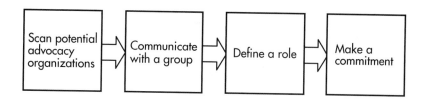

FIGURE 17–2.   Steps in becoming an advocate.

ilies can understand and utilize the information provided, and they want professionals to share their own ideas and help create new services by providing technical assistance to develop and manage the organization.

A great disappointment to leaders of child advocacy groups is working with professionals who do not recognize the expertise of parents. Parents believe that they know their children's problems and needs the best. In training families in advocacy, leaders disabuse parents' common belief that professionals know everything. Wise leaders help families see that professionals too have good days and bad days and that professionals work long hours in a stressful and emotionally draining occupation. Mental health professionals choose their profession because they care as deeply about the health of children as families, but some do not understand parents or care for them in helping ways. Families need respect for their expertise, and professionals need partnership and appreciation.

Working Together for the Best Interest of the Child

Anyone working with child advocacy groups quickly realizes that child advocates are not a group of tame parents; they are determined to secure better services for their children. For professionals who are aware of how few children receive needed psychiatric treatment, the moral obligation to become involved with an advocacy group is apparent. Without sufficient advocacy, funding of services will continue to be inadequate; research will continue to lag far behind that dedicated to multiple sclerosis, cystic fibrosis, or other less prevalent disorders; discrimination will still exist in insurance, in social relationships, and in other life areas; and the right to a childhood free from immense pain and misery will not be secured.

Just before his death, Martin Luther King Jr., responding to the enormous difficulties and challenges of the civil rights movement, quoted the Talmud: "You are not obliged to complete the task—but neither are you free to desist from it." In the struggle to secure adequate mental health services for children and adolescents, families alone do not have the resources or energy to build a better system; they need the energy, passion, skills, and resources of professionals to advocate beside them for needed changes to the system. Everyone benefits in a collaborative partnership between advocacy groups and caring professionals. Most importantly, such partnerships benefit the ultimate goal of a child having a stable life of decent quality in an environment that provides an opportunity for his or her life to have meaning.

■ ADVOCACY AND TECHNICAL RESOURCES ON THE INTERNET

The Internet has recently become the premiere channel of communication for advocacy groups and professionals. Many advocacy groups and resources are quickly and easily found on the World Wide Web. E-mail is a popular way to communicate for most advocates and professionals. Listed below are several major child psychiatry advocacy organizations and information resources on the Internet that professionals can use for researching and connecting with groups. The list is not meant to be complete or all-encompassing but to provide basic resources that can be used to improve both practice and relationships with families and advocates.

Advocacy Organizations

The American Academy of Child and Adolescent Psychiatry (http://www.aacap.org) advocates for children and adolescents with "developmental, behavioral, emotional, and mental disorders." The academy works with other advocacy groups such as NAMI, the National Mental Health Association, and the Federation of Families for Children's Mental Health. Membership is open to child and adolescent psychiatrists, other physicians such as pediatricians, and medical students with an interest in child and adolescent behavioral disorders. The organization's Web site features an outstanding online library of informational fact sheets primarily targeted to parents.

The Autism Society of America (http://www.autism-society.org) is devoted to increasing public awareness about autism and the day-to-day issues faced by patients, their families, and the professionals with whom they interact. It publishes a newsletter, holds an annual conference, and sells books related to autism.

The Child and Adolescent Bipolar Foundation (http://www.bpkids.org) is relatively new, formed in 1999 in response to the lack of understanding and focus on bipolar disorder in children and adolescents. The primary purpose of this parent-led group is educating and raising awareness among the public about early-onset bipolar disorder.

Children and Adults With Attention-Deficit/Hyperactivity Disorder (http://www.chadd.org) is a national organization that offers information and support to families and adults with attention-deficit/hyperactivity disorder (ADHD) and gives guidelines to parents and others interested in starting support groups. It advocates for research, corrects misunderstandings about ADHD, holds an annual conference, and provides an online store of educational resources for consumers, families, and providers.

NAMI (http://www.nami.org), a leading advocacy group for families and persons with severe psychiatric disorders, advocates for services and research for adults, adolescents, and children at the federal, state, and local levels. It has a school-based educational curriculum and a number of support programs for parents. The NAMI Information Helpline connects parents and others to local and state affiliates: 800-950-NAMI (6264).

The Federation of Families for Children's Mental Health (http://www.ffcmh.org), a parent-run organization with affiliates in each state, focuses on children and adolescents with emotional, behavioral, or mental disorders and on families' needs. The federation is currently developing a training curriculum focusing on family involvement in treatment. The federation publishes a newsletter and holds regular conferences.

The National Mental Health Association (NMHA; http://www.nmha.org) welcomes volunteers, who can choose from advocacy activities at national, state, and local levels. Professionals have always played a role in NMHA activities, serving communities across the nation. A large nonprofit organization with a particularly strong child and adolescent mental health focus, NMHA provides public education and sponsors Mental Health Week. Its Web site includes a comprehensive section on children's mental health advocacy. NMHA is involved in many coalitions advancing mental health in legislative arenas.

Informational/Technical Resource Organizations

The Center for Effective Collaboration and Practice (http://cecp.air.org) is a collaboration of the U.S. Department of Education and the Center for Mental Health Services (CMHS) of the Substance Abuse and Mental Health Services Administration (SAMHSA), U.S. Department of Health and Human Services. Its Web site includes a section titled "Promising Practices in Children's Mental Health" (http://cecp.air.org/promisingpractices) that provides information about excellent systems of care for treating child and adolescent psychiatric disorders and includes a strong focus on family collaboration articles.

The Web site of Georgetown University Center for Child and Human Development (http://gucchd.georgetown.edu/index.html) in Washington, D.C., includes multiple links to useful publications, conferences, training opportunities, and other Web sites organized by topic. The center is funded by CMHS/SAMHSA. For technical assistance, call 202-687-5000.

The Research and Training Center for Children's Mental Health (http://rtckids.fmhi.usf.edu) at Louis de la Parte Florida Mental Health Institute of the University of South Florida focuses on children's mental health services research, particularly evidence-based practices. It produces many useful publications and recommends improvements for child and adolescent mental health systems. It is jointly funded by the U.S. Department of Education and CMHS/SAMHSA.

The Research and Training Center on Family Support and Children's Mental Health (http://www.rtc.pdx.edu), based at Portland State University, is similar to the center at the University of South Florida.

The University of California, Los Angeles (UCLA) School Mental Health Project–Center for Mental Health in Schools (http://smhp.psych.ucla.edu) is one of two technical assistance centers (the other is listed below) focusing on school-based mental health services. The center at the UCLA is funded by the Health Resources and Services Administration and CMHS/SAMHSA. The center provides online technical assistance, continuing education and in-service training, and many useful articles and guides for school mental health services.

The East Coast counterpart to the UCLA School Mental Health Project described above is The Center for School Mental Health Assistance (http://csmha.umaryland.edu), located at the University of Maryland School of Medicine in Baltimore.

▌ CONCLUSIONS

Opportunities abound for professionals and child advocates to work together for the best interests of children and adolescents with mental illness and their families. History indicates that much good can flourish when collaboration is viewed as transpiring among those bringing equal skills, resources, and energy to the table. The future is bright for such collaboration and cooperation to bear lasting benefits to all involved.

▌ REFERENCES

Education for All Handicapped Children Act of 1975, Pub. L. No. 94-142

Individuals With Disabilities Education Act Amendments of 1997, Pub. L. No. 105-17

Joint Commission on the Mental Health of Children: Crisis in Child Mental Health: Challenge for the 1970s. Bethesda, MD, National Institute of Mental Health, 1969

Juvenile Justice and Delinquency Prevention Act of 1974, Pub. L. No. 93-415

Juvenile Justice and Delinquency Prevention Reauthorization Act of 1993, Pub. L. No. 102-586

Knitzer J: Unclaimed Children: The Failure of Public Responsibility to Children and Adolescents in Need of Mental Health Services. Washington, DC, Children's Defense Fund, 1982

Paul Wellstone Mental Health Equitable Treatment Act, S. 486, H.R. 953, 108th Cong. (2003)

Teplin LA, Abram KM, McClelland GM, et al: Psychiatric disorders in youth in juvenile detention. Arch Gen Psychiatry 59:1133–1143, 2002

Torrey EF: Out of the Shadows: Confronting America's Mental Illness Crisis. New York, Wiley, 1997

White House Conference on Child Health and Protection, 1930, U.S. National Archives Records Administration, Dwight T. Eisenhower Library, Abilene, Kansas

▌ SUGGESTED READINGS

Coursey RD: Serious mental illness: the paradigm shift involved in providing services and training students, in New Directions in the Psychological Treatment of Serious Mental Illness. Edited by Marsh DT. Westport, CT, Praeger, 1994, pp 123–140

Friesen BJ: Parents as advocates for children and adolescents with serious emotional handicaps: issues and directions, in Advocacy on Behalf of Children With Serious Emotional Problems. Edited by Friedman RM, Duchnowski AJ, Henderson EL. Springfield, IL, Charles C Thomas, 1989, pp 40–41

Griffin-Francell C: Advocating for seriously emotionally disturbed children and their families: an overview. J Child Adolesc Psychiatr Ment Health Nurs 6:33–37, 1993

Griffin-Francell C, Domenici N: The role of family education. J Clin Psychiatry 54 (suppl):31–34, 1993

Hospital to Home Focus Group: Working With Professionals: Personal Advocacy. Seattle, WA, King County Interagency Coordinating Council, 1992

Knitzer J: Children's mental health: the advocacy challenge, in Advocacy on Behalf of Children With Serious Emotional Problems. Edited by Friedman RM, Duchnowski AJ, Henderson EL. Springfield, IL, Charles C Thomas, 1989, pp 18–23

Lefley HP: An overview of family professional relationships, in New Directions in the Psychological Treatment of Serious Mental Illness. Edited by Marsh DT. Westport, CT, Praeger, 1994, pp 166–185

McElroy E: Introduction, in Children and Adolescents With Mental Illness: A Parents Guide. Edited by McElroy E. Kensington, MD, Woodbine House, 1988, pp 93–110

PART

IV

Outcomes and Future Directions

18 TRANSITIONS FROM INSTITUTIONAL TO COMMUNITY SYSTEMS OF CARE

Dean X. Parmelee, M.D.

Peter Nierman, M.D.

In this chapter, we describe closings of state-operated psychiatric facilities in two states in the final decade of the twentieth century, provide information on the political and fiscal issues prompting the closings, and describe how child mental health clinicians forged plans to ensure that children and families would not lose out on needed services. Each state is unique, but all states have the potential to dismantle mental health services for children *or* to create services that go beyond the managed care nonsense of drive-through crisis intervention and stabilization. As child mental health clinicians assumed leadership, they prevailed on the political processes to take risks in developing a system of care, managed to anticipate changes, and synthesized disparate resources for the desired end product. Follow-up on what has happened since the closings is also presented.

■ CASE ONE: VIRGINIA

Background

In 1991, the Virginia Department of Mental Health (VDMH) was ordered to significantly reduce its budget because of the state's revenue shortfall. It was decided that $5 million could be saved by closing the Virginia Treatment Center for Children (VTCC), a 32-bed inpatient facility on the campus of Virginia Commonwealth University (VCU), a state medical school in Richmond. The children from the area could be cared for at a state adult facility 30 miles south or at another children's facility a 2-hour drive west. Some employees could transfer to either of these facilities, depending on their seniority; many others would be laid off. The director of VTCC (Robert Cohen, Ph.D.), a direct appointee of the VDMH, had to develop plans for employee layoffs and patient transfers on a closing date that was just months from the decision announcement. The medical director (Dean X. Parmelee, M.D.), a medical school faculty member on contract for services to the state, was requested to assist with the clinical issues of the transition period.

However, both clinical administrators decided to catalyze the university's interest to instead acquire the facility (prime real estate) and instigated political pressure from families, legislators, professionals, and community mental health workers from the region. The chair of the university's department of psychiatry was instrumental in building support within the medical school and the university for making a deal with the VDMH; the deal would carry low financial risk and would maintain the integrity of the training and education programs originating from the treatment center. About 60 days before the expected closure, the governor announced that VTCC would not be closed and that plans were in progress for the VCU Medical Center to operate the facility. Although there was much relief from the successful acquisition of the center, the facility's leadership knew that major challenges loomed. For example, it would not be easy to achieve the financial goals of the medical center in a very competitive managed care environment (i.e., with the center no longer receiving state funds).

Crucial Points

The VTCC leadership began an appraisal of how the treatment center could do well in a managed care environment, still serve a community mental health population, and build a stronghold for academic child psychiatry in a huge medical school complex. Within 18 months of the proposed closing, a number of changes were initiated.

Continuum-of-Care Services

No longer under the VDMH, VTCC could go beyond providing 32 inpatient beds and could create a more comprehensive program to include the following:

• *Outpatient services:* To include contracts with regional community mental health centers (CMHCs) for the psychiatric components.

- *A day hospital program:* To be responsive to the requests of managed care companies to help children make the transition from acute care more quickly.
- *A residential care program (20 beds):* To fill an expanding need for children who need much more than a few days of acute care (which is all managed care will allow).
- *An acute care program (12 beds):* To focus on evaluating and stabilizing patients and then refers them within the new system of care or back to a local community provider.
- *Home-based services:* To be provided in conjunction with community clinics. CMHCs struggle to create and maintain therapeutic settings in regular homes and in foster care or group home arrangements. This program helps CMHCs develop programs for children who are using the acute care and other institutional care services heavily but who could be managed in the community.

Changing Attitudes Within and Without

All VTCC staff members had to adopt a consumer-first attitude, wherein the consumers are the patients, patients' families, third-party payers, community mental health clinics, school systems, social service agencies, and juvenile courts. No longer could there be the notion of "us against them." The center had a product to offer that could be purchased either at the center or elsewhere. It took several months for everyone on the staff to realize that his or her paycheck depended on happy customers. No longer could the staff see themselves as the poor, underfunded, besieged state hospital; they had to be the best full-service psychiatric facility for children in the area.

The community mental health clinics were accustomed to sending children to the center, where they would stay until they got better. The VTCC had to develop a new relationship with the clinics wherein the center's staff were partners or consultants in helping the clinics with their most troubled cases. This change was difficult, because the center could no longer keep children awaiting disposition. When children became clinically stable, they had to be discharged, and the community became obliged to assume a new level of responsibility. This forced the issue of building a continuum of care in the community, something that is often more developed for adult services than for children's.

▌ CASE TWO: ILLINOIS

Background

In 1997, the Illinois Division of Mental Health (IDMH) decided to close the last state-operated psychiatric hospital for children and adolescents serving the greater Chicago metropolitan area. The decision was fueled by comparisons of lengths of stay in private versus public facilities and shifts toward providing more care in the community. Potential obstacles to the closure included 1) the impact on local and statewide labor relations, 2) the fact that some children might fall through the cracks if the resultant system was not seamless, and 3) the possibility of the closure process becoming politicized when it was submitted to the state legislature for approval.

The principals involved in the planning and execution of the process (all of whom were specialists in child mental health) kept the needs of children and families paramount. They were convinced that the principles of a managed care approach could ensure quality care within a community continuum and could allow the state to redirect valuable finances to areas of need. No additional funding was available, given the $660 per diem cost at the state facility compared with a negotiated rate around $425 at area private hospitals, where stays were dramatically shorter. The projected savings were $9 million.

Crucial Points

The network charged with ensuring a transition to the new model of care established an executive team after the closure announcement in March 1997. The network manager, a child and adolescent psychiatrist (Peter Nierman, M.D.), and other child mental health specialists on the team were deemed critical for establishing credibility with the varied constituencies involved: parents of mentally ill children, private hospitals and private psychiatrists, CMHC directors and line staff, and children's rights advocacy groups. The executive team produced the vision of an enhanced community-based system of care with careful but appropriate scrutiny of the use of the inpatients' money.

Early Discussions of Closure

The immediate obstacle of labor opposition was acknowledged. The facility had more than 225 employees, most of whom were labor union members. The union had joint bargaining responsibilities for more than 20,000 state employees statewide. The closure would have implications for labor-management relations if the union leadership interpreted it as a sign that the state was advancing a plan to close all state-operated hospitals. The prospect of layoffs would stiffen opposition to the closure. The labor relations concerns were eased when it was determined that positions for all staff members were available at other regional facilities. Every employee was offered a position at either an adult mental health facility or a facility for the developmentally disabled.

Creating a System of Care

The executive team deemed a seamlessly functioning network to be essential. It was readily apparent that to the child and adolescent CMHC system in the Chicago area, which was receiving approximately $15 million yearly via grants and contracts from the IDMH, an addition of several million dollars a year *could* greatly enhance services. Selecting the private hospitals for the project required a process of site visits that took several months. At each site visit, the network manager formally inspected the facility, discussed anticipated terms of the contract, and conferred with the clinical staff on treatment philosophy. The discussions during these visits always addressed the following:

- Staffing patterns
- Use of restraint and seclusion
- Use of psychotropic medications
- Awareness of community systems
- Internal policies to address allegations of patient mistreatment

Hospital administrators were asked to complete a survey in which they provided written responses regarding the following topics:

- Service capacity, security, and safety concerns
- Behavioral-level systems
- Multiple-language and cultural competency
- Areas of subspecialty
- Partial hospitalization programming
- Twenty-three-hour observation bed availability and other distinguishing characteristics

A final contract between a selected hospital and the network included language describing the steps for parents and guardians to access IDMH hospital services for their children. To be eligible for funding, parents or guardians with no means to pay for necessary mental health services would be required to have their child evaluated by a community screening agent (a qualified mental health professional), who would determine whether appropriate community-based services were available and appropriate as an alternative to hospitalization. The contract also contained language that mandated a close working relationship between the community screening agents and the hospital staff. Hospitals were required to specify child and adolescent psychiatrists who would be responsible for treatment of youths under this program and to invite community agents to staff meetings, make proper notification of upcoming discharges, and complete discharge summaries within a week of discharge. The contracts also mandated that hospitals hold regular administrative meetings with the community teams to address communication difficulties, working relationships, or the complex needs of some children and families. Children with extraordinary needs consistent with neuropsychiatric disorders, first psychotic experiences, potential seizure activity, and genetic or metabolic disorders could receive additional tests and services (such as computed tomography scans, magnetic resonance imaging, electroencephalograms, and investigatory blood tests) with authorization from the network medical director. Hospitals agreed to notify the network within one working day of all new admissions. The first utilization review conference would occur on the fifth working day after admission, and weekly conferences would be held thereafter. Clinicians would be asked to justify continued hospitalization in accordance with published network criteria. This review would be conducted by a registered nurse under the supervision of the network medical director.

The network maintains an extensive database on all children and adolescents admitted through the program. The executive team decided that evaluating clinical outcomes was as crucial as evaluating cost savings. Information collected on all inpatients includes vital statistics and demographics, hospital and community agency contacts, and relevant clinical data. To obtain data on transitions to less intensive levels of service, 30- and 120-day continuity-of-care follow-up telephone surveys to community programs were completed on every case. Parents were asked to complete a consumer satisfaction survey after their child's discharge.

The network adopted principles of the Child and Adolescent Service System Program to help identify objective measurements that reflected quality. A Total Quality Improvement model was employed to address the functions of monitoring and quality control. The basis for determining areas of focus for quality assurance was a combination of consumer input, the guiding principles, and selected service transition points.

Addressing the Political Process

The final potential obstacle to be confronted was the unpredictable nature of the political process (i.e., how would the privatization of mental health services be interpreted by the final arbiters of the state budget?). Discussions were held with area experts in the field of child and adolescent psychiatry to hear their concerns and garner their support. Some key community providers and trade organizations that were viewed as industry leaders were brought into planning discussions. Key political figures and legislative liaisons were consulted to prepare for possible appearances before legislative committees. A formidable consensus by stakeholders was developed using both the proposed clinical outcomes (better care for more children) and the potential for cost reduction, with more money being available for community-based services.

The hospital closure made possible an unprecedented transfer of funding to community services. The transition plan called for all funds previously dedicated to the hospital to be maintained for child and adolescent mental health services in the network. The planned expansion of the child and adolescent community service system promised to infuse over $9.5 million in new funding and to increase service capacity by nearly 65% throughout the network.

One initial budget shift was to transfer nearly $1 million to the Department of Corrections, Juvenile Division. This funding reflected an estimate of the annual expense for services dedicated to youths who had been admitted to the facility from juvenile correctional facilities. The Juvenile Division was able to hire additional clinical staff at youth centers to perform psychiatric diagnoses and psychological assessments and to administer more intensive treatments to incarcerated adolescents.

❚ UPDATES ON THE TRANSITIONS

Virginia Program

VTCC remains wholly owned and operated by the VCU Health System. Its array of inpatient, outpatient, and community-based services continues to develop. The undergraduate and postgraduate training in several mental health disciplines has been enriched by the evolution of services and responsibilities. The center is paying for itself financially, although it must constantly fight to hold on to the resources it has in a health care system with declining revenues. The program has managed to do this by carefully managing expenditures and maximizing revenues. For example, better day rates were negotiated with insurance companies and some state agencies because of the quality of reports generated and because of the closing of many other regional child and adolescent centers. VTCC has striven to provide specialized services within its mission as a teaching hospital and community resource, to develop a specialized trauma focus within its residential unit, to provide more community-based services within schools, and to diminish disparities in access to mental health care for the children it serves.

Illinois Program

The Illinois program continues to flourish. In the year before the hospital was closed, 225 youth were admitted, with an average length of stay (ALOS) of

56.5 days. The statistics for 1999 indicate considerable increases in the numbers of children under 13 (N=103; ALOS=11 days) and in the numbers of adolescents (N=338; ALOS=11.6 days) with significantly shorter lengths of stay after being served in hospitals. Of the children and adolescents served at 16 participating hospitals, 58% were eligible for Medicaid. The total network cost was less than $2 million, or $425/day—well under the cost of providing state hospital services. Through community funding enhancements made possible by the closing of the state hospital and reapportionment of its allocation, a flowering of new services in office or home assessment or treatment occurred:

- Newly funded programs served 219 youngsters through 5,675 purchased service units (i.e., a documented clinical contact with a child).
- Previously underfunded programs served an additional 650 youngsters.
- Outreach and family support services to families residing in Chicago public housing served 500 families with 25,000 service units ($100 per service unit).
- Multidisciplinary assessments were received by 250 clients.
- Local CMHC services were expanded by increasing the availability of a child psychiatrist and by providing case management and coordination; liaison with juvenile justice, police, and welfare agencies; and consultation to local schools.
- The $1,700,000 allocated to this program resulted in service for 715 clients.
- The largest allocation ($1.8 million) expanded the screening, assessment, and support services (SASS) program; the program includes a parent empowerment program that functions as a consumer-operated network to assist all families of children being served.
- Of the 1,325 clients evaluated for hospital services, 67% were referred for intensive community services directly through SASS, and 33% were referred for hospitalization.

Thus, besides the savings realized from the closing, a considerable increase in the quantity and quality of individualized services has resulted.

∎ CONCLUSIONS

In these two case examples, child and adolescent clinician-administrators can be seen orchestrating some novel responses to the customary state approach of eliminating services for children and adolescents to save money. In the Virginia case, the leadership group designed a model of care with the old facility serving as the hub in a wheel. In the Illinois case, the leadership used the emerging managed mental health care model to allow the closure of a state facility without losing the most intensive level of care as inpatient care was shifted to the private sector and nonhospital-based services were greatly expanded. This project has remained very successful, and the prescreening procedure is being adopted in New York City and Rhode Island.

Both the Virginia and Illinois programs creatively developed a full system of care to meet the needs of the public sector and the families in need of psychiatric services. They provide models for the immediate future of delivering psychiatric and other mental health services within the community.

▌ SUGGESTED READING

Nierman P, Lyons J: State mental health policy: shifting resources to the community: closing the Illinois State Psychiatric Hospital for Adolescents in Chicago. Psychiatr Serv 52:1157–1159, 2001

19 INNOVATIVE COMMUNITY INTERVENTION PROGRAMS

Lawrence A. Vitulano, Ph.D.

John R. Holmberg, Psy.D.

Donna S. Vitulano, M.S.W.

The practical necessities of community-based work are described and illustrated throughout this book. Meaningful collaborative efforts in community-based work have resulted in cutting-edge programs that have recently emerged and are in the process of being developed. In this chapter, we describe several ongoing community-based intervention efforts at the Yale University Child Study Center in New Haven, Connecticut. Although these are not the only programs under development, they illustrate issues germane to community-based work and directions for innovative programming to address critical needs. The programs described are the Family Support Services (FSS) program, Yale Intensive In-Home Child and Adolescent Psychiatric Services (IICAPS), the Program for HIV-Affected Children and Families, and the Child Development–Community Policing (CD-CP) Program.

The Child Study Center's FSS program was based in part on in-home programs developed in the 1970s. The Homebuilder Program in Tacoma, Washington, was one of the first to provide in-home services in the community (Nelson 1990). That program was operated by a nonprofit organization with the intent of averting out-of-home placement through provision of short-term, home-based therapy and case management by a master's-level clinician. The treatment intensity and duration were typically 5–18 hours a week for 1–6 months. Home-based treatment employing this basic model has been widely used across the country (Bogenschneider 1996). Adnopoz and associates (1996, p. 1076) provided a listing from Kaplan's (1986) earlier review of community-focused home-based programs that had been proved to be effective with children of families with multiple problems. In that review, seven key features were identified: 1) the family is viewed as the patient or unit of treatment, although the child is the identified patient; 2) services are provided to the family in their home; 3) it is assumed that change is possible when family strengths, not weaknesses, are pursued; 4) services are time limited; 5) the focus of service is on keeping families together and preventing unnecessary foster placements; 6) services are intensive, and case loads are low by design; and 7) concrete services (i.e., food, shelter, and safety) and advocacy (i.e., case management) are provided.

▋ CHILD STUDY CENTER INNOVATIVE PROGRAMS

Family Support Services Program

At the Child Study Center, Woolston and colleagues (1998) implemented two in-home programs that take the Homebuilder model further. In the FSS programs, they focus attention on integrating the multiple systems (e.g., from intrapsychic to intrafamilial, and from community to broader social systems) that affect the functioning of any one child-family unit. FSS is a 24-hour, in-home voluntary program developed to help families with children who are at imminent risk of being placed out of the home (Adnopoz et al. 1996). The FSS program, developed in 1985, has a unique treatment team approach. The FSS model integrates the features identified by Kaplan (1986) but also provides intervention based on a team approach. The clinical team is composed of a clinician (e.g., psychologist or master's-level clinician) and a trained layperson who functions as a family support worker.

The family support worker is a critical component of the treatment approach. These workers are often recruited from identified neighborhoods and are typically in tune with the heartbeat (e.g., the trends, lifestyles, resources, language uses, and political issues) of the community. Whenever possible, one or both members of the treatment team are assigned to cases based on their multilingual abilities, to allow for the provision of services in the family's primary language. The family support worker is an equal treatment partner and often serves as an effective role model with whom the client family can identify (Adnopoz et al. 1996). As treatment partners, the FSS team collaborates with the multiple agencies and systems affecting the family and shares responsibility with those agencies and systems for critical case coordination and collaboration.

Although fiscal and time constraints on resources are considered, the FSS model also emphasizes the importance of conducting a thorough initial assessment of strengths and needs of the family and of planning for discharge from the first contact. Although most programs do so implicitly, the FSS model also explicitly focuses intervention on the best interests of the child. Implementing services in the family home provides an opportunity to intervene with the possibility of reduced resistance, observe interactions in vivo, and gain a sense of neighborhood and community factors that would otherwise be intangible in a clinic-based intervention.

Yale Intensive In-Home Child and Adolescent Psychiatric Services

IICAPS represents the latest derivation of the in-home approach. Using the FSS model and the theoretical developments emerging from wraparound-services models (e.g., VanDenBerg and Grealish 1996), IICAPS adapts the in-home approach to families who face the difficult task of coping with having a child or children with significant psychopathology or serious emotional disturbance. Families working with the IICAPS program have typically experienced more than their fair share of contact with social service agencies such as police departments, probation offices, detention centers, specialized schools, and inpatient psychiatric hospitals. The wraparound model adapted by IICAPS includes several important components. One is the weekly treatment rounds staffed by the clinical teams, supervisors, and coordinators (including the psychiatrists, psychologists, social workers, mental health clinicians, and experts in public health). Although the concrete aspects of reviewing the current clinical situation are of primary concern, the hypothesized aspects of clients' difficulties (i.e., developmental, psychodynamic, and systems aspects) are analyzed, and the treatment components are discussed. The clinical team also provides an arena for clinicians to provide mutual support, which is much needed due to the high intensity of home-based work. Another unique aspect of IICAPS is the emphasis among the coordinators on establishing and maintaining strong relationships and open lines of communication. These lines are both bottom-up (i.e., extending from case workers to administration) and top-down from leaders of other social service agencies (e.g., department of justice, social service agencies, and public schools) to families. Coordinators at IICAPS are also actively involved in policy decisions at the local, state, and national levels. Most policy-level interventions involve volunteering time to establish dialogues with legislative committees; serving on advisory boards; and facilitating meetings with heads of other social service agencies to coordinate services, identify unmet needs, and develop collaborative solutions to system-level difficulties. Finally, IICAPS is now in the process of implementing a system of data collection to be conducted at first contact and repeated at termination. This system will enhance the initial clinical assessment process with formally collected measures and will also be used to evaluate outcomes of the interventions.

Program for HIV-Affected Children and Families

A third program at the Child Study Center is the Program for HIV-Affected Children and Families. This child-focused, family-centered program provides services in clients' homes and communities. The clinical team approach that is used, based on a model of relationship, contributes to the uniqueness and creativity of this therapeutic intervention for children and families. The clinical team offers a range of services, including family therapy, individual psychotherapy, parent guidance, psychological testing and evaluation, psychiatric consultation, and support groups for children and caregivers, as well as case management, client advocacy, and permanency planning. The dynamic interaction of these services is based on the psychosocial and cultural needs of the child within the family and provides for a comprehensive treatment model.

The tremendous physical and psychosocial demands placed on those parents diagnosed with human immunodeficiency virus (HIV) infection and acquired immunodeficiency syndrome (AIDS) often create a difficulty or a reluctance to seek assistance both for the parents and for their children. Families affected by HIV live in a climate of stigma, secrecy, and loss. Emotional struggles permeate their daily lives and complicate new issues that are already difficult. Permanency planning, disclosure, and various socioeconomic challenges create ongoing change and crises. Children developing under these strains have many unanswered questions and experience unexplained events, which often lead to anxiety, fear, and depression. Intervention with these families is a multilevel treatment incorporating mental health care, support, and advocacy. Bringing the services into homes and communities provides accessibility and personal attention for families that are too overburdened and isolated to benefit from traditional programs.

To illustrate the program, the case of a 12-year-old Latino boy and his 8-year-old sister demonstrates how the children's and the family's psychosocial needs are met through the home-based clinical treatment model:

The boy was referred by his mother's case manager for individual counseling when family members, caring for him while his mother was hospitalized with AIDS, became distressed by some of his annoying behaviors. The mother had refused earlier counseling referrals for the children, but she now agreed to accept help for her son. The boy verbalized frequent frustration at school, as well as allusions to suicidal ideation. Although the mother was dying of AIDS, she maintained the desire to keep an environment of secrecy, refusing to disclose her diagnosis to her children. The inability to discuss the situation led to feelings of anxiety for the boy and sadness and depression for the girl. Although no services were requested initially for the 8-year-old girl during the intake process at the home, it was apparent that she too was greatly affected by her mother's illness. She had a flat affect, and her curiosity with the clinician's presence and her apparent desire to become involved with her brother's intervention seemed to indicate a need for some individualized adult attention. She was provided a program clinician for weekly home-based play psychotherapy. Clinical treatment for both children focused on helping them work through feelings of anger and frustration about changes in their lives due to their mother's health concerns. Other family services included preparing the mother to begin to discuss her impending death with the children. She was thus able to help them prepare for their anticipated grief and eventual loss. Because the mother had drafted a will and had identified family members to take custody of the children after her death, permanency planning was addressed by helping the mother feel comfortable in verbalizing this plan to her children. When members of the extended family came from the mother's homeland to help care for her and the children, family treatment was initiated. Treatment efforts engaged the relatives in the children's current lifestyle and helped them to think about the children's needs for the future. Collaboration with medical and social service agencies assisting the family was an important component of the intervention. An emphasis on the children's needs and necessary collaborative efforts by providers was reinforced. Advocacy efforts for the 12-year-old boy led to school consultation regarding psychosocial and cultural issues affecting his performance and achievement. Short-term bereavement counseling was a focus after the mother's death. Final services linked the family with resources in the mother's homeland, to which the children and relatives returned.

Child Development–Community Policing Program

In the final program to be considered, a very different but equally intense type of clinical work is being conducted in the New Haven community. During 1991, due to increasing concerns about the particular burden that exposure to violence was placing on children's development in the community, the CD-CP Program was developed. The program, based on the application of sound developmental principles, began as a collaboration between the Yale Child Study Center and the New Haven Department of Police Services (Marans et al. 1995, 2002). It is the outgrowth of several early meetings about shared concerns for children among clinicians and police. The CD-CP

Program involves attempts to reorient police officers in their interactions with children and consequently to better utilize the psychological role of police as providers of a sense of security and benign figures of authority. This collaboration allows mental health clinicians the opportunity to play a more significant role in the lives of children and families exposed to violence in the community, in the home, and in schools.

Although police officers come in daily contact with children who are victims, witnesses, and perpetrators of violence, they generally do not have sufficient professional training, time, or other resources necessary to meet these children's psychological needs. Conversely, clinic-based mental health professionals may be professionally equipped to respond to the children's psychological distress but have little opportunity to do so. Unfortunately, traumatized children are rarely seen in outpatient clinics (if they are seen at all) until months or years later, when chronic symptoms or maladaptive behavior brings them to the attention of parents, teachers, or the juvenile courts. This situation results in the loss of valuable opportunities to intervene at the moment when professional contact could be most useful and to provide both immediate stabilization and bridges to a variety of helpful ongoing services.

Currently, the CD-CP Program provides a range of training and consultation services in the community, including having a senior clinician on call 24 hours to be available to officers, children, and families who are directly involved in violent incidents. At a weekly conference, cochaired by police officers and clinicians, cases are presented, information is shared, and treatment plans are developed. It is regularly attended by senior clinicians, police officers, staff members from the probation and protective services departments, and any other individuals (e.g., the beat officer and the child's former therapist) who are able to contribute to the care and planning of the specific cases being discussed. In addition, clinicians meet weekly for discussion and supervision of this intense collaborative work that often requires immediate action and involvement in horrific, traumatic situations. Over the years, we have found that this work cannot be done alone. It necessarily takes an interdisciplinary approach with team members who are mutually supportive and available to work together at a moment's notice. The nature of this work often requires more than one or even two clinicians to be involved in the treatment of families with multiple children.

The CD-CP training approach is collaborative by necessity. Police train clinicians and clinicians train police in their respective procedures, responsibilities, and interventions. The best interests of the child always guide the work. On tours of duty, police officers spend many hours taking clinicians on ride-alongs, explaining and showing how they work, and then spend just as many hours in the classroom teaching clinicians about police administration, procedures, tactics, and other essential matters. Concomitantly, clinicians offer an introduction to the theories of development that guide their work, with an emphasis on a practical approach to understanding and helping children and families. For example, police officers find it quite helpful to understand why babies often cry when separated from their caregivers or why adolescents must be so challenging on the streets in front of their peers.

The CD-CP model has been replicated in several cities across the United States and in Europe. In the past 4 years alone, the New Haven police have referred over 1,000 children and their families who have experienced violence, as well as hundreds of children who have committed serious violent offenses. These children are usually seen within minutes of the police response to scenes of violence and tragedies, such as murders, stabbings, beatings, fires, drownings, and gunfire. The children and their families have been seen individually and as part of larger groups in their homes, at police substations, at schools, in their neighborhoods, and within the Child Study Center. Specialized outreach teams have been established for victims and child witnesses of domestic violence as well as for juveniles in detention. Specialized outreach programs have been instituted for high-risk children, both in the schools (for children exposed to gang and other related forms of violence) and through the courts (for gateway delinquents who are first-time offenders and are at risk of developing more chronic patterns of antisocial or other maladaptive forms of behavior).

Overstimulation and excessive levels of stress often threaten a child's newly consolidated and most recently attained developmental capacities. The subsequent regression is especially compromising for a child whose development is already fragile. However, it is essential that one's assumptions about a child's possible traumatization not be derived solely from the facts of the violent event but rather from the meaning attributed to the event by the child. To determine the best interventions to use, clinicians must learn about the child's experience of the external events in the context of his or her inner life. Above all else, clinicians must continue to be good and careful listeners.

Children's exposure to violence may precipitate a host of responses that reflect the powerful convergence of internal and external dangers derived from both the past and the present that are mediated by the degree of support and availability of the family. Unfortunately for far too many children in this country, the violent horrors that should belong only to the world of the child's most primitive fears and terrors are materialized in real-life experiences. As a result, the basic feelings of safety and security that are essential to the child's developing sense of competence and mastery are severely undermined. However, symptoms that follow these traumatic experiences may also introduce a small window of opportunity for informed proximate interventions that can help to identify and untangle the various webs of danger and that consequently can help a child return to a more normal path of development.

■ CONCLUSIONS

Innovative community interventions require a collaborative spirit and the will to make positive changes in the direction and structure of programs. Such successful intervention programs are based on the following:

- The integration of rich clinical experiences
- Flexible programming that reaches out into the community
- The application of sound psychological and systems theories
- A focus on the whole family
- The dedication of a committed and well-trained clinical team
- Ongoing supervision that is open, practical, and instructive

In this chapter, we describe several community programs that have been developed and adapted to become effective treatment approaches. By integrating clinical experience and sound theory, and with undying dedication, the clinical teams have been successful in reaching the children and families who are most in need of services through the application of creative and innovative interventions. The principles epitomized by these programs need to be kept in mind when developing special initiatives in the public sector, but such programs and principles reflect only the current stage of development in what needs to be an ongoing evolution for mental health providers.

■ REFERENCES

Adnopoz J, Grigsby RK, Nagler SF: 105 Multiproblem families and high-risk children and adolescents: causes and management, in Child and Adolescent Psychiatry: A Comprehensive Textbook, 2nd Edition. Edited by Lewis M. Baltimore, MD, Williams & Wilkins, 1996, pp 1074–1080

Bogenschneider K: Family related prevention programs: an ecological risk/protective theory for building prevention programs, policies, and community capacity to support youth. Fam Relat 45:127–138, 1996

Kaplan L: Working With Multi-Problem Families. Lexington, MA, Lexington Books, 1986

Marans S, Adnopoz J, Berkman M, et al: The Police–Mental Health Partnership: A Community-Based Response to Urban Violence. New Haven, CT, Yale University Press, 1995

Marans S, Murphy RA, Berkowitz SJ: Police–mental health responses to children exposed to violence: the child development community policing program, in Child and Adolescent Psychiatry: A Comprehensive Textbook, 3rd Edition. Edited by Lewis M. Philadelphia, PA, Lippincott Williams & Wilkins, 2002, pp 1406–1416

Nelson K: Populations and outcomes in eleven family based child welfare programs, in Family Preservation Services: Research and Evaluation. Edited by Wells K, Biegel D. Newbury Park, CA, Sage, 1990, pp 72–91

VanDenBerg JE, Grealish EM: Individualizing services and supports through the wraparound process: philosophy and procedures. J Child Fam Stud 5:7–22, 1996

Woolston JL, Berkowitz SJ, Schaefer MC, et al: Intensive, integrated, in-home psychiatric services: the catalyst to enhancing outpatient intervention. Child Adolesc Psychiatr Clin N Am 7:615–633, 1998

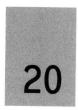

20 FUTURE DIRECTIONS

Theodore A. Petti, M.D., M.P.H.

Child psychiatry and allied mental health professions have a well-deserved reputation for collaboration and innovation, as demonstrated by their efforts in the public sector. The Olmstead decision (*Olmstead v. L.C.* 1999) will be a further catalyst for developing public-sector psychiatry; the decision mandates the provision of community services in facilities caring for four or fewer persons. Additional change can be expected as attention to the site of care for severely and persistently ill adults progresses to considering the needs of psychiatrically ill children and adolescents—that is, those diagnosed with serious emotional disturbance (SED). Local counties and other public entities are struggling to find appropriate placements for youngsters with disruptive or psychotic behavior, for whom community living has been problematic and has been considered unrealistic. Following the principles of the Child and Adolescent Service System Program (CASSP), programs funded by the federal Center for Mental Health Services provide opportunities to demonstrate how positive outcomes can be expected by extending the mandate of the *Olmstead* decision to juveniles.

▌ THE FUTURE IS NOW

Current initiatives and developments in community child and adolescent psychiatry are essential for extending the reach and efficacy of needed care. Considerable innovation is thriving in the community mental health arena, and more innovation can be expected in the future:

1. The Dawn Project, begun in Indiana in 1997, created new family-based services in the community to serve such children in conjunction with a private community agency. The program provides family-centered residen-

tial care. The children can either sleep at home or stay overnight in the facility. The parents are called for direction when the children require discipline at the facility. Policies emanating from the *Olmstead* decision may increase the pressure to provide more of these coordinated community mental health services. Systems of care will likely flourish as their effectiveness is demonstrated (see Pumariega and Winters 2003).

2. The settlement in an Arizona class-action lawsuit (*J.K. v. Eden* 2001) concerning children covered by Medicaid may hasten the process of providing needed psychiatric services elsewhere. The settlement is expected to do the following: reform a statewide managed care system for children's mental health, force adherence to 12 guiding principles (Bazelon Center for Mental Health Law 2001), and change the behavioral health care system in the direction of the CASSP initiative. The settlement requires increased funding; training for staff in assessment, planning, and delivery of services; and hiring specially trained staff to work with specified populations. Future suits (e.g., from the Bazelon Center for Mental Health Law) and national news headlines in this area can be expected.

3. Blending public and private resources is gaining momentum as programs throughout the United States focus on wraparound structures to meet the needs of identified youngsters with psychiatric difficulties. The numbers of outcome evaluations are increasing, and further increases can be expected during the coming decade. Formal and informal systems of care that blend or decategorize funds (i.e., eliminate categorical restrictions for use) will be developed and maintained. These systems will improve the levels of communication and collaboration between various agencies and both the value and effectiveness of public monies spent in the interest of children and adolescents with SED and those at risk of becoming ill. Legislation in some cases and regulations in others will be needed to decrease or eliminate the administrative barriers to successful implementation of such systems.

4. Advocacy and consumer groups, professionals, and professional organizations will join to promote federal initiatives to keep these promising initiatives alive and growing. Academic centers and state mental health agencies will develop continuing education programs about evolving mental health and family law. Practitioners, administrators, attorneys, students, and trainees of mental health and related disciplines will learn to use case and legislative law for the benefit of their patients and their families. Families can be expected to participate at all levels of service delivery, policy development, and evaluation as the field moves to a family and community focus for care and decision making. Family members will

increase their involvement as key players in these ventures. Greater emphasis will be placed on community activity, including variants on treatment in residential and hospital settings. More care will be delivered in schools and juvenile detention centers. Mental health professionals will better understand the operation of these systems and will develop skills for active collaboration with fellow professionals working within them. Training community mental health workers (CMHWs) and families about reimbursement within the public system and how to gain access to such funding is crucial to successful functioning of any system of care. Interdisciplinary efforts will be critical, as will engagement at some level in the political process.

5. Public-sector professionals will be expected to collaborate with primary care physicians, nurses, teachers and other school personnel, day care workers, and those working in welfare and juvenile justice sectors. Tasks include early awareness and detection of psychiatric illness (i.e., risk factors for mental illness and the use of screening and rating scales and other assessment or monitoring instruments), consultation and collaboration for disseminating knowledge about the principles of therapeutic behavior management, and facilitating communication with parents on mental health–related issues.

6. Greater emphasis on early intervention and prevention of disability will accompany efforts to treat those with SED (e.g., Chang et al. 2003). Professional organizations will assist CMHWs to keep abreast of current legislation and regulations concerning the care and treatment of children and teenagers with medical and psychosocial illness. These organizations will have greater interaction with advocacy groups to educate the general public, lobby government for needed programs, assist patients and their families in gaining access to support programs—such as the State Children's Health Insurance Program; Temporary Assistance for Needy Families; and the old standby, Early and Periodic Screening, Diagnosis, and Treatment—and ensure that those programs are being funded and provided. With the evolving insights gained from research in the areas of attachment and cognitive development, work with children from early infancy through adolescence and early adulthood will be taking place in multiple settings tailored to the needs of individual children and their families (Casey 2004). CMHWs treating adults and families with severe or chronic psychiatric illnesses should be required to identify all children whose parents show any suggestion of dysfunction or symptoms of emotional distress and refer those children for evaluation and treatment.

7. Technology will be utilized more effectively and comprehensively in diagnosis and treatment. The Multimodal Treatment Study of Children

With Attention-Deficit/Hyperactivity Disorder (MTA Cooperative Group 2004) and the Treatment for Adolescents With Depression Study Team (March et al. 2004) and their offshoots provide clinicians with improved tools for assessment and evidence-based treatment (EBT) of the most prevalent psychiatric disorders of childhood. Similar efforts can be expected for the treatment of other childhood psychiatric disorders. Interdisciplinary efforts to identify EBT in psychosocial and psychopharmacological areas will facilitate integrating these developments into the field (see Burns and Hoagwood 2002). Neuroimaging will frequently be employed in the diagnosis and assessment of the more severe and persistent psychiatric disorders and ultimately in evaluating the efficacy or effectiveness of specific or bundled treatments. Telemedicine—via special telephone lines, satellite communication, and the Internet—is expanding access to research and clinical updates, allowing public agencies to communicate with tertiary-care clinicians for rapid consultation and initiation of EBT. New buildings will require hard wiring and satellite capability for bidirectional information exchange.

Community and public-sector workers are becoming comfortable with terms such as *efficacy* (short-term effectiveness of a particular treatment) and *effectiveness* (sustained or positive effect over longer periods of time). Effectiveness studies will be conducted in community settings and away from purely academic centers. EBTs will be evaluated for their value in the actual community as opposed to the academic and research world, perhaps by employing networks of clinicians outside the arenas of academic and large urban hospitals to conduct real-world studies of the short- and long-term costs and benefits of existing and developing medications (March et al. 2005); psychosocial therapies; and multimodal, multisystemic approaches to assessment and treatment. As the knowledge base for assessment and EBT expands, CMHWs, policy makers, and administrators will need to be familiar with practice parameters or guidelines from professional organizations such as the American Academy of Child and Adolescent Psychiatry (http://www.aacap.org) and the National Institutes of Health (http://www.nih.gov). Treatment algorithms will expand in number, level of acceptance, and use.

8. Systemic approaches to service delivery in the community will proliferate. Wraparound services and multisystemic therapy (see Burns and Hoagwood 2002) are two important and increasingly employed models of providing services for youngsters and their families who need intensive and long-term psychiatric care. Likewise, reliable and valid instruments for documenting actual services delivered or received will be used to advocate for improved legislation and regulations.

With the continued shift toward community assessment and treatment and family-focused care, access to services becomes critical. Lowering barriers for minority families to receive mental health care and related services and developing a better understanding of the cultural context within which a family or group within the community is living will become a major responsibility of CMHWs. Isaacs-Shockley and associates (1996) provided a succinct approach to this issue. CMHWs will learn to value diversity in the general culture and will craft prevention and treatment strategies that increase cultural competence in the system (e.g., performing a cultural self-assessment, understanding the dynamics in which cultural differences affect service delivery and effectiveness, and incorporating the insights gained). Principles for accomplishing these tasks were nicely demonstrated by Podorefsky and associates (2001).

The practice of community mental health care calls for progressively greater involvement in the public-policy arena to influence allocation of sparse funds and requires a sufficient knowledge base to allow comfort when testifying or advocating for a particular position, policy, or direction. Lurie (2000) cited the recent report by the Institute of Medicine detailing three factors that hinder clinicians from providing high-quality care within the current safety net:

a. The disproportionate costs borne by clinicians from serving a growing number of uninsured patients
b. The erosion of traditional subsidies maintaining the health care safety net
c. Adverse effects resulting from the rapid shift to Medicaid managed care

As a response, networks of public-sector allies can be expected to share access to relevant data sets and to advocate for improved funding and services via the Internet. Learning to gain access to these treasures of information takes time and effort but is worth the expenditure. Disseminating this information in usable packets to the public and to agency staff will increase both advocacy efforts and effective, efficient delivery of services.

Areas of service delivery are being affected by policies with potential for benefit or harm. For example, prior authorization has become a means for cost containment, but it can also be a means of improving disease management or case management. Knowledgeable personnel can play a major role in shaping the form and role for such structure and policies, including how these structure and policies are developed and implemented. Policy in disease or case management can have impacts on all levels of prevention. For example, appropriate assessment and treatment of preschool children who have symptoms of attention-deficit/hyperactivity disorder can prevent such children from receiving inappropriate treatment with stimulant medication or can ensure that correct diagnoses are made and that required psychosocial and biological interventions are provided.

9. Likewise, discontinuity of services in the transition to adulthood by adolescents with severe and persistent mental illness has caused many of these youths to relapse and fall through the cracks. A major challenge will be to construct a system and train case managers and clinicians to identify and begin early planning for these youngsters when the transition to adulthood clearly will need to be supported by coordination and collaboration with multiple agencies, the family, and the youngster. Efforts to allow successful transitions toward independence should build on federal and state regulations to ensure appropriate care without placing undue burdens on the family, the clinician, or the agency (Clark and Davis 2000). Reaching out to educational, vocational rehabilitation, welfare, religious, and charitable organizations should allow such a network and system to be created and maintained for individual teenagers and their families. Two key pieces of federal legislation will play pivotal roles in the expansion of services in this process: 1) the Americans With Disabilities Act (P.L. 101-336) and 2) the Individuals With Disabilities Education Act (P.L. 105-17). Both set expectations for the care of persons with psychiatric disorders. Familiarity with these laws will be helpful when advocating for appropriate mental health services.

▌ CONCLUSIONS

These are truly interesting times, in which advances in technology and clinical approaches serve as the backdrop for some real opportunities to provide improved services and more effective interventions earlier in the course of children's mental illness. For example, an economic downturn offers the chance to try innovative strategies in the structure and function of community mental health services. Likewise, a growing economy with budget surpluses offers the potential of supportive funds to provide intensive and extensive levels of early intervention and prevention for children, adolescents, and their families who are at risk for serious and persistent mental illness.

This book details some of the creative ideas, programs, and concepts taking place in the community mental health arena. We hope readers have gained a better sense of the opportunities for the good work and satisfaction available from working in or consulting to community agencies—and of how readers, as mental health professionals, might be able to participate. We also hope that readers better understand how mental health and related systems function, about the professionals who work in those systems, and about options for assisting the system in reaching its potential. We wish each reader the very best of success as he or she decides to take the journey into the universe of community mental health for children and adolescents.

▌ REFERENCES

Americans With Disabilities Act of 1990, Pub. L. No. 101-336

Bazelon Center for Mental Health Law: Principles for the Delivery of Children's Mental Health Services. Washington, DC, Bazelon Center for Mental Health Law, 2001. Available at: http://www.bazelon.org/jkprinciples.html. Accessed February 23, 2005

Burns BJ, Hoagwood K: Community Treatment for Youth: Evidence-Based Interventions for Severe Emotional and Behavioral Disorders. New York, Oxford University Press, 2002

Casey BJ (ed): Developmental Psychobiology. (Review of Psychiatry Series, Volume 23; JM Oldham and MB Riba, series editors). Washington, DC, American Psychiatric Publishing, 2004

Chang K, Dienes K, Blasey C, et al: Divalproex monotherapy in the treatment of bipolar offspring with mood and behavioral disorder and at least mild affective symptoms. J Clin Psychiatry 64:936–942, 2003

Clark HB, Davis M: Transition to Adulthood: A Resource for Assisting Young People With Emotional or Behavioral Difficulties. Baltimore, MD, Paul H Brookes, 2000

Individuals With Disabilities Education Act Amendments of 1997, Pub. L. No. 105-17

Isaacs-Shockley M, Cross T, Bazron BJ, et al: Framework for a culturally competent system of care, in Children's Mental Health: Creating Systems of Care in a Changing Society. Edited by Stroul BA. Baltimore, MD, Paul H Brookes, 1996, pp 23–39

J.K. v Eden, CIV 91-261 TUC JMR, United States District Court for the District of Arizona (2001)

Lurie N: Strengthening the US health care safety net. JAMA 284:2112–2114, 2000

March J, Silva S, Petrycki S, et al: Fluoxetine, cognitive-behavioral therapy, and their combination for adolescents with depression: Treatment for Adolescents With Depression Study (TADS) randomized controlled trial. JAMA 292:807–820, 2004

March JS, Silva SG, Compton S, et al: The case for practical clinical trials in psychiatry. Am J Psychiatry 162:836–846, 2005

MTA Cooperative Group: National Institute of Mental Health Multimodal Treatment Study of ADHD follow-up: 24-month outcomes of treatment strategies for attention-deficit/hyperactivity disorder. Pediatrics 113:754–761, 2004

Olmstead v L.C., 527 US 581, 138 F3d 893, affirmed in part, vacated in part, and remanded (1999)

Podorefsky DL, McDonald-Dowdell M, Beardslee WR: Adaptation of preventive interventions for a low-income, culturally diverse community. J Am Acad Child Adolesc Psychiatry 40:879–886, 2001

Pumariega AJ, Winters NC (eds): The Handbook of Child and Adolescent Systems of Care: The New Community Psychiatry. San Francisco, CA, Jossey-Bass, 2003

INDEX

Page numbers printed in **boldface** type refer to figures or tables.